breatheology

Stig Åvall Severinsen

breatheology
the art of conscious breathing

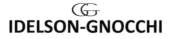

IDELSON-GNOCCHI

breatheology
© 2012, 2010 Stig Åvall Severinsen

Editors: Mark Colberg Goldsmith
         Constance Kampf
         Brittany Trubridge

Graphical design and layout: Mark Colberg Goldsmith

Cover: Casper Tybjerg
Photo p. 70: Appreciation of the exhibition *Bodies*
Photo p. 99, 126 and 257 Morten Bjørn Larsen
Photo p. 137 Per Hallum
Photo p. 138 Dan Burton
Photo p. 174 Mallar Chakravarty

Set in Calibri

© 2012, Revised edition
© 2010, 1. edition

ISBN 1-928649-34-3

BlueConsult

www.blueconsult.biz
www.breatheology.com

© 2012 Published by Idelson-Gnocchi Publisher Ltd., Subsidiary Publisher Division of
IDELSON-GNOCCHI Srl - Editori dal 1908 - **www.idelsongnocchi.it**
Sorbona • Grasso Morelli • Liviana Medicina • Grafite • Idelson Gnocchi Ltd.
Via M. Pietravalle, 85 - 80131 Naples, Italy - Tel +39-081-5453443 - Fax +39-081-5464991

Idelson Gnocchi Publisher, Ltd. - **www.manualoffreediving.com**
1316 King's Bay Drive, Crystal River FL 34429, USA - Tel. +1 352 361 9585 - Fax +1 561 207-7132

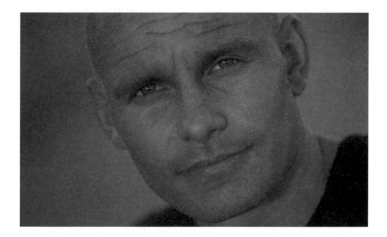

Stig Åvall Severinsen (born 1973) is a four time World Champion freediver. Freediving consists of diving deep or long while holding your breath. He holds a Master's degree in biology (2001) and a PhD in medicin (2007) from the University of Aarhus, Denmark. During the last decade he has practiced and investigated the beneficial effects of breathing and breath holding on body and mind.

Through his company BlueConsult, blueconsult.biz, and his international web community **breathe**ology, he offers courses and lectures on efficient breathing and mental training.

Join his community at www.breatheology.com and get access to free breathing tutorials today.

Contents

Appendix

*To Trine, who has helped me breathe and hold my
breath over the years
&
To Damian, who stopped breathing
much too early*

Preface

Unconscious breathing

"Yahweh God shaped man from the soil of the ground and blew the breath of life into his nostrils, and man became a living being"
GENESIS 2:7

Your life is lived between two breaths – your first inhalation and your last exhalation.

Each day you breathe between 20,000 and 30,000 times. This amounts to roughly 10 million breaths each year and one billion breaths in a lifetime. You are probably good at breathing, but it is actually very likely that you are not using your lungs to their full capacity. This is a shame because if you do not utilize every breath you are waving goodbye to extra energy in your daily life.

Most people are not very conscious of how they breathe. In particular, poor breathing habits are common in modern times. When was the last time you took a deep and slow breath and thought closely about the intimate relationship between your breath, your body and your mind?

By consciously taking hold of your breathing, you have a unique opportunity to change and strengthen both your body and mind. Our incredible organism is capable of transforming itself to a degree that science has not believed possible. Thus, recent research shows us that the human lung is capable of increasing its size through training, and that positive thoughts can, in fact, affect and rejuvenate your brain. If you learn how to improve your physical and mental capacity, your general health and your chances of living a long life will improve.

It may seem odd that many people are ignorant about such a natural thing as breathing. Both animals and children breathe deeply down into their "stomach" and thereby utilize the lungs optimally. However, for busy people, this is more the exception than the rule. This unfortunate fact is mainly determined by social and cultural trends due to the hustle and bustle of everyday life, which has distanced us from our body. All in all, this leads us to completely forget the calm and deep breathing we were given at birth. Life is rushed and often we forget to listen to our bodies.

Unlike, for instance, heart rhythm or digestion that only a few people can control, anybody can learn to control their breathing. Naturally, this will not reduce the stress or the workload in your life. However, gaining more oxygen in the organism and a more relaxed nervous system can help you become better at managing the pressure and unpredictability of life. All you have to do is remember to consider your breathing.

Indeed, breathing is exactly what this book is about. I hope to initiate you into the enormous potential that mind control and conscious breathing can bring to your life in order to manage stress and increase your daily energy level. When your lungs become stronger, you have a better "filter" in your body, you will be able to absorb more oxygen and gain more energy in every cell, while at the same time your body will be more able to more efficiently eliminate or expel metabolic waste products.

Become aware of your breathing

There are two points at which your body, and often your mind, is under extreme pressure: during "extreme" or ultimate athletic performance and when facing a life-threatening illness. By becoming familiar with the reactions of the body in these extreme situations, you can come to understand how conscious and efficient breathing habits can contribute to more positive energy in your everyday life.

Since my childhood, I have loved water, nature and sports. Today, I have integrated all three of these into freediving at a professional level. Freediving is about holding your breath under water. You can achieve this most easily when you are relaxed and in control, which has always felt natural to me when I dive. I consider freediving an adventurous sport – not an extreme sport – but I readily admit that some people find it extreme. Nonetheless, I have selected safe and efficient breathing techniques influenced by freediving but modified so that anybody can use them. As you learn conscious breathing techniques, you will find the benefits relevant to your daily life.

Since I was a child, I have spontaneously used several of the conscious breathing techniques, and during the last ten years, I have begun to use some techniques with more reflection—both when working towards world records in freediving and in my everyday life. To optimize my performance, I have practiced yoga regularly. The central goal of yoga is to control your breathing to strengthen your body and gain greater peace of mind. The knowledge of different yoga techniques is an essential tool in gaining optimal efficiency of your breathing.

As opposed to mind control techniques, which so to speak, work from the inside – from mind to body – this book deals primarily with techniques that work from the outside in by focusing on breathing – from body to mind. It is easy to concentrate on breathing and whether you are young or old, sick or healthy, efficient breathing techniques are safe and easily exercised habits that can be used by anyone.

These breathing techniques are not new but rejuvenated wisdom about breathing from ancient practices such as yoga. For example, **pranayama** *– a traditional aspect of yoga, is composed of two Sanskrit words. The first,* **prana**, *meaning life force, and the second,* **ayama**, *meaning control. If we understand breath in terms of life force, there is a connection between controlling your breath and controlling your life force. This key concept from pranayama is one of the influences on the discussion of body and mind as connected through efficient breathing, which is part of the basis for this book.*

I view life from a holistic perspective and believe that body and mind influence each other respectively. In the same way, I believe that people should live in harmony with nature rather than dominating it. I continue to be fascinated by living organisms, and curious to know about their design and function. Studying biology, which in Greek means "the science of life," was a natural course for me to take – what can be more interesting than life itself? Consequently, I earned a PhD in medicine. My scientific background stems from the natural and health sciences. Therefore, during the book I refer to the benefits of breathing exercises and breath control on body and mind – be it concerned with sports, illnesses or any other cause.

Breathe efficiently

Each chapter in this book will show you how you can breathe more efficiently and the advantages you can gain through conscious changes in your breathing habits. Since each chapter highlights different themes in relation to breathing, these can be read individually, but it may be more rewarding to read the chapters in succession.

> *In chapter one, **Restless breathing**, you will be able to recognize the effects of unconscious and uneasy breathing in everyday life. This chapter focuses on ways in which calm and conscious breathing can prevent and control stress, and how weight can be managed through breathing. In addition, the influence of mind power and your diet on your physical and mental well-being will be examined.*

> *Chapter two, **Normal breathing**, describes how breathing works, and how it affects your body. When you more fully understand how your body and your nervous system are organized, you can more easily change any potential bad habits. In this chapter, you will learn how your breathing is regulated, and how you, by way of being conscious about your breath, can activate the soothing part of your nervous system and increase your daily well-being and health.*

> *Chapter three, **Trained breathing**, provides an introduction to yoga, giving not only the historical and philosophical background on a holistic basis, but also valuable exercises that you can use to attain a more serene body and mind. Understanding how breathing bridges the gap between your physical and mental self, you can learn to understand the finer nuances of breathing – one of the central elements of yoga.*

> *In chapter four, **Sustained breathing**, the many advantages of breath holding will become clear. Even though you may not think about it in your daily life, pauses in your breathing are quite natural and often spontaneous. In pranayama (controlled breathing) breath holding is particularly important. When you realize how the body and mind both change and become stronger, you will also understand how conscious breathing techniques can be applied in self-development and in your daily life.*

> *Chapter five, **Powerful breathing**, describes the many advantages that breath holding as well as breathing techniques, can add to sports – both for everyday exercise and elite athletes. Many of these stem from the freediving universe, however, they are excellent for everyday use. In addition, I describe experiments with the heart, brain and lungs, which provide scientific examples for why a greater awareness of breathing is so important. This chapter provides techniques to improve your performance and results in your fitness routine.*

> Chapter six, **Therapeutic breathing**, pinpoints how you can boost your health through conscious and efficient breathing. Should you be ill, this chapter offers valuable advice as to how you can work towards recovery and minimize your disease. Furthermore, efficient breathing is also a potent aid for preventing illnesses.

> Chapter seven, **Soothing breathing**, describes how you can relieve pain by strengthening the connection between body and mind both through calm and attentive breathing as well as through positive thinking, imagery and meditation. By shifting your focus to your breath, the pain will seem less intense and a more regular heartbeat will soothe and nourish the body.

I believe that everybody ought to have a basic knowledge of life saving first aid. Thus I have added a brief appendix on artificial respiration and heart massage.

Once you have expanded your knowledge of breathing techniques in relation to a particular theme, you can immediately begin with the techniques for efficient breathing. Following each chapter you can find a set of exercises that are easy to perform and at the same time efficient. Do not be fooled by their apparent simplicity. The more you practice, the more you will grow aware of the complexity of each exercise. The breath is very refined and exciting to work with because new layers of your inner self are constantly revealed. Each time you have an "aha" experience during training, you may learn a little more about yourself – and about other people too. This is exactly why it is so fun and fascinating to work with the connection between body and mind.

If you think that it is probably necessary to perform breathing exercises or meditation for months or years before you experience marked results, you are mistaken. From my own experience and from people I have taught, I know that significant changes can happen in a matter of minutes, hours or days. A recent scientific study actually showed that body-mind training combining relaxation, conscious breathing, imagery and mindfulness meditation revealed measurable changes in subjects following 5 days of 20 minute daily training. The participants showed less tension, were in a better mood, had an improved immune response as well as significantly fewer stress-related hormones in their blood. You will find examples of these body-mind exercises in this book and hopefully my concept of breatheology – the learning and teaching about how we breathe – will encourage you to start your own adventurous learning experience. If you want to expand your knowledge or get free video

*demonstrations of the exercises presented in this book, you can visit my
international community – www.breatheology.com.*

*I do not promise that you will become happier with conscious and effi-
cient breathing, but I guarantee that you will become more cheerful and
have more energy and greater reserves in your everyday life.*

Enjoy!

*Stig Åvall Severinsen
Aarhus, Denmark
August 1st, 2010*

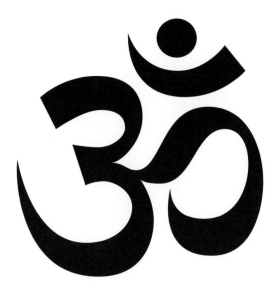

Part I

Unconscious breathing

Part I looks at how our breathing can become uneasy or stressed from a hectic everyday life. Furthermore, it examines normal unconscious breathing patterns and pinpoints criteria that you can use to examine your own habits - good as well as bad ones. This is important in order to get a deeper understanding of how your breathing works and affects your body and mind.

This knowledge will give you an understanding from which you can develop more conscious breathing habits, which will be thoroughly examined in part II.

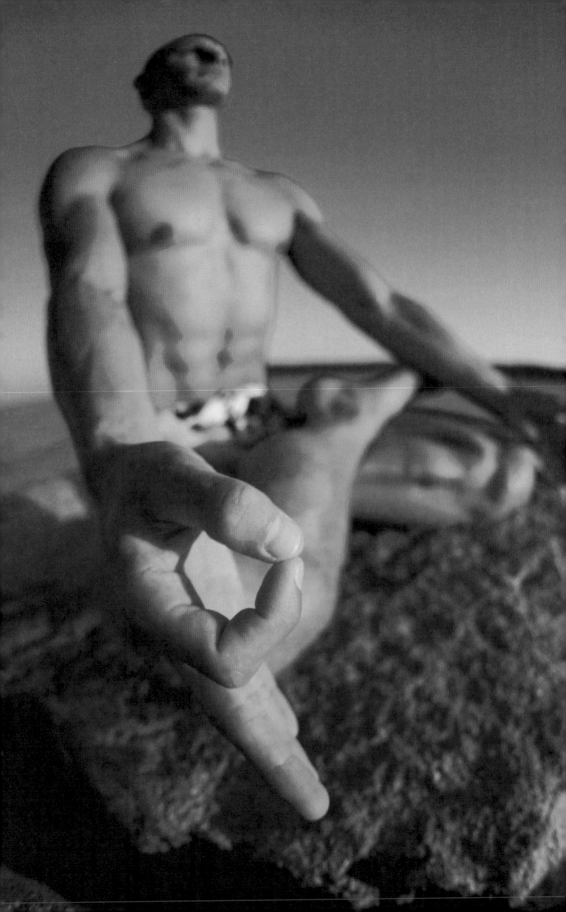

Restless breathing

A hectic everyday life

The daily breath

Your breathing is a perfectly accurate and honest barometer for your emotions. You can feel for yourself how stress affects the ease and pace of your breathing – especially the way you inhale. If you become aware of this strained condition, you can "heal" yourself simply by taking a few conscious breaths - soft, deep and slow. Instantly, you will discover that a deep peace settles in your mind. Conscious breathing is quite elementary and extremely efficient. Taking soft deep breaths should provide you with an immediate sense of how you can manage the restlessness in your body and your galloping thoughts by simply controlling your breath.

> "Live your own life, for you will die your own death!"
> Roman proverb

The amazing part of becoming aware of your breath is that, in time, the nervous system will become conditioned, which will make your unconscious breathing deeper, calmer and more harmonious. The point of training your breath is to create a stronger and more stable nervous system and thereby an advantageous method of breathing – your own new and natural breath. In this way, your natural unconscious breath will be beneficial in everything you do - since your breath influences your body from even the finest nerve fibers to all your organs, your hormone production, and even your thoughts. In addition, during the night you will be able to harvest the fruits of your new breath in the shape of deeper and more tranquil sleep.

When I take the bus, train, airplane or stand in an elevator, I notice how people breathe because it reveals a lot about their state of mind. It is also interesting to observe how people breathe when they are about to attempt something mentally or physically challenging.

The more you learn about the finer details in breathing, the more you can learn about people by observing them from a short distance. When I train or coach others the first thing I look for is the depth, frequency and variation in their general breathing pattern. Next, I examine deeper and finer layers of their breathing. For example, facial expressions, body language and muscular tension are important parts of the human puzzle, which come together before my eyes.

Through the years, I have developed an intuitive sense that often targets a person's balance between physical and mental faculties. Particularly, when I ask people to hold their breath or train them in breath holding exercises, I learn a great deal about their mental condition and capacity. In addition, people learn much about themselves. This training is quite simple but also effective and certainly one of the best forms of self-development and self-management, simply because you cannot "cheat" others nor yourself, as it cannot be faked.

Exactly for this reason, breath holding is one of the best methods to learn relaxation and mind control, even though it can be a demanding and challenging process. I will not claim that I can see colors or auras streaming out of people, but I can certainly sense some kind of energy, and I can readily relate to how people are doing and sense their thoughts, because I have been there many times myself.

Body tension can also be revealed through breathing and breath holding, not only where tension is located but also how much tension a person has built up inside. Tension is often located in the shoulders, face and neck. I usually say, "your neck has to be as soft as butter", and it often helps straight away.

Different color nuances and complexities of the skin are also part of my observation because they reveal the blood circulation and oxygen content of the blood. I regularly write down the time I believe a person can hold his or her breath, and most of the time I am not far off. It is an amusing little game (usually for myself), but the fascinating and interesting part of it is to see how far you can move people within a short time. Tiny adjustments or corrections often yield big results, and I let my intuition and pocket philosophy have free scope. No holds are barred, so the challenge is to find the right methods for the person in question. The point is not that everybody has to become world champion freedivers, but it makes me happy when my students become "world champions" in breathing correctly, because I know how much this will be of help to them for the rest of their lives in relation to using both body and mind.

The ability to relax "on command" and overcome or completely avoid stress and the accompanied improved mental control and confidence are gifts that help in all parts of life. I have clearly observed this whenever I have been working with elite athletes, business managers, retired people, children, disabled, or people who are ill.

"Your breathing exercises and meditation opened a new world to me. The act of closing out the world, and being in both myself and my breath is completely unique. Never before have I experienced such calmness and balance. I have used this process daily ever since. Both in sports and my training – where I concentrate on getting oxygen to all the muscle fibers – and also when I am under pressure at work and need to make quick decisions which can have big economic consequences. Instead of breathing with the upper part of my lungs, I lean back and breathe way down to my legs – and then I move on. Breathing is a remarkable tool to keep stress at bay."

Charlotte Eisenhardt, 35
Construction manager at NCC Construction Denmark A/S

Fresh air

Consider how you use or misuse your breath every day. Breathe properly and open the window for a few minutes at your office or in your home, so fresh air can reach your lungs.

New research from Japan and Korea actually shows that fresh air can increase mental effectiveness by 10 – 20%. People simply become better at carrying out practical tasks and their memory improves. Thus, it is worth paying attention to the indoor environment that surrounds you, such as temperature, moisture level, number of green plants, dust etc. Who has not experienced the feeling of being heavy and tired in body and mind after a long day at a stuffy office? It wears down your health and private life as well as the economy of your workplace. As a manager, it may also be comforting to know that by simply adjusting environmental conditions, staff health and productivity can be raised.

A study performed by DTU – the Danish Technical University in Copenhagen, showed that this is also true for Danish elementary school students. On average, students working in poor environmental conditions lose the equivalent of a complete year of education in terms of productivity. Consequently, there is a price for not considering indoor environment, fresh air and proper breathing on both health and learning.

At times, it can be quite appropriate to hold your breath. If behind the exhaust of a bus or truck, it is the most natural thing in the world for me not to breathe. Some may think this is stretching it a bit far, but when you consider the amount of particle pollution we are exposed to every day in cities, it is not totally crazy. In the United States, the organization Clean Air Task Force (CATF) released the "No Escape" report in 2007,

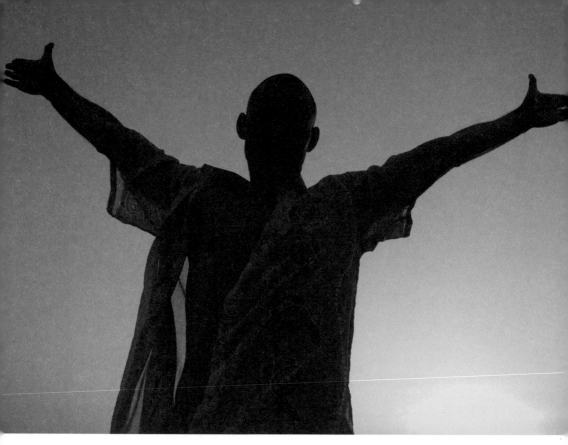

Fresh air and light increases your daily energy level.

estimating that diesel fumes kill about 21,000 people each year in the US, and further stating that at least 70,000 Americans each year have their life shortened by diesel exhaust particles. Furthermore, scientists link serious health impacts such as asthma, disruption of normal heart rhythm, heart attacks, strokes and lung cancer with diesel fumes.

Although we might smile when we watch Japanese and Chinese people on television wearing masks in the streets of larger Asian cities, it may not be that silly at all.

The revealing breath

Our breath is so finely tuned, that it can reflect our personal health, and thus reveals which factors in our environment affect us negatively. Any sensible person knows that a large amount of alcohol, greasy foods, inactivity and daily stress do not improve health.

"When the breath is irregular, the mind wavers; when the breath is steady, so is the mind. To attain steadiness, the yogi should restrain his breath."

HATHA YOGA PRADIPIKA

We have to dig deeper to understand the reason why such an unhealthy and unnatural life style has become the norm. Perhaps, it is the most important question of our time and the greatest mystery. We must understand which imbalances in our body, mind and soul draw us in the wrong direction – and why! Our breathing reflects our life situation, our feelings, and allows us to consciously enter the deepest recesses of our complex mind. As I previously mentioned, your breath is a personal barometer of your condition which reveals whether you are thriving or not, but it demands that you listen.

Inscribed in the old Temple of Apollo are the words "Know Thyself". Breathing is the best tool to accomplish self understanding because it bridges the gap between your body and your mind.

We can utilize our breath to influence our daily physical and mental health to a greater extent than many think. The obvious next step is taking a closer look at how you can manage stress through breathing.

What is stress?

About 50 years ago no one "suffered" from stress. This is not because stress did not exist, but because the term had not yet been coined.
In order to understand and manage stress, a clear sense of what the term covers is needed. The word stress is often associated with something unpleasant, undesirable and dangerous. It is problematic that the word functions as a black box filled with all kinds of "evil" because there are also plenty of good and positive forms of stress.

"Without stress, there would be no life."

HANS SELYE

The inner natural balance in humans is termed *homeostasis*. The word originates from Greek (*homeo*: same/similar and *stasis*: stable), and describes an organized physiological equilibrium in an open system, i.e. a body or a cell. Everything that draws the body away from equilibrium is stress. At the same time, processes which restore equilibrium are also stress. One might say that stress is an elastic process which compensates and adjusts, and this regulatory process has recently been named "*allostasis*". *Allo* comes from Greek and means "variable". The range of possible states which surrounds homeostasis is thus caused by allostatic mechanisms. These mechanisms maintain stability through change.

Let us take a typical situation: if you suddenly run a couple of meters, an allostatic response will immediately start. You breathe more quickly and your pulse increases – you are experiencing stress. This kind of stress is both positive and necessary because it compensates for the increase in oxygen consumption and blood supply. As soon as you stop running, your rate of breath, your pulse and your blood pressure drop again. This allostatic response restores equilibrium because a constantly elevated pulse is no longer useful to your body. Thus, through "stress", equilibrium is maintained.

Two key points can be learned from this example. First, moderate, temporary and effective stress is positive at the right place and time. It gets your system in an alert state and ready to meet new challenges. However, when the stress is prolonged and too extreme, it becomes negative. The body gets worn down and deteriorates - a condition we know as chronic stress. Chronic stress is dangerous, undesirable and probably the kind of stress that you think of, when you hear the word. This condition is also known as allostatic overload – the system has simply been strained beyond capacity like a rubber band that snaps. The allostatic mechanism originally designed to protect you now becomes destructive.

The second important point you can learn from this example of a short run is that you can influence your stress through breathing. This is useful knowledge because your breath is an incredible allostatic tool designed to regulate your stress. Calm and controlled breathing will bring your exhausted body and brain back to the starting point – homeostasis in perfect balance, a glassy lake on a summer's day.

The mechanisms behind stress

Stress results from circumstances that affect your inner balance. Positive stress is about facing resistance and challenges, thereby creating healthy growth and protecting your system. This is the way you build up a muscle – bit by bit. In the same way you can exercise the brain and keep it tuned. In contrast, negative stress exhausts and destroys, as a result the system simply "goes off the rails".

But what does stress look like, and what activates it in the body? Stress uses the neuroendocrine system, which implies that it functions through nerve messages affected by our hormone-producing glands. Stimuli from the outside as well as the inside can initiate stress. The brain and body work together to react to changes – physical, psychological or both.

Psychological stress, like physical stress from an inflicted injury or just a run, can be divided into various temporary states. These states encompass conditions such as mild depression, anxiety, anger and even hostility. Other psychological stress factors such as conditions at work, in the home, your personal financial situation or daily life can be referred to as psychosocial stress and are often chronic in nature.

Whatever the reason for stress, your reaction to it is predominantly governed by two complex hormone systems. These systems secrete *adrenalin* and *cortisol*. Adrenalin works fast and is the "survival hormone" of the body. If, for instance, you are about to fall, drop something or become very scared, you can feel an adrenalin rush in your body. Cortisol, on the other hand, has a delayed secretion after a stressful event. Thus the two hormones are secreted at different moments in relation to the stress level. Both cause wear and tear on the body and mind if they are constantly present in high concentrations in the blood. If the hormone systems are under pressure for an extended period, they can eventually "run wild" - leading to stress, depression, psychosis or other mental disorders in addition to physical illness.

The amount of stress needed to activate these response systems vary from person to person. Animals, as well as humans, that have been raised in an insecure and unpredictable environment elicit a higher stress response to mild stressors than those raised in stable and secure environments. People who suffer from chronic stress have a stronger reaction to mild stress. These individuals will often be more depressed or aggressive, since their *serotonin* levels are low. Serotonin is a hormone which keeps us in a good mood. This is also true of patients suffering from depression, which in many instances can be caused by stress. In some of these cases, antidepressant medicine is prescribed to help raise the serotonin level in these patients.

It is not surprising that so many people suffer from stress in this rapidly changing world. In our rushed modern society, we are extremely rational and analytical on a high intellectual level, but the complexity and unpredictability of life stresses and frustrates us. Mobile phones go off all day long and increased demands of productivity at work, in the home, on holiday and in sports clubs generally cause stress because our own and others expectations of ourselves can be unrealistic and unreasonably high. When these psychological stress factors are combined with inefficient breathing, unhealthy diet and too little exercise, the result is a vulnerable system in which sometimes "a single straw can break the camel's back".

Since your lifestyle or a high workload can be difficult to change, it is beneficial to look for other ways of managing your stress. Luckily stress can be managed in many other ways and breatheology offers a path that I have found effective in my life. The workload in itself does not necessarily lead to stress. However, unpredictable moments that spark the hormone faculties of the brain do. If you adopt a different strategy in your reaction and utilize the creative and intuitive capacities, many problems can be seen as interesting challenges and new solutions suddenly begin to appear. It is a useful and workable way of dealing with your stress, and fortunately you can train techniques that stimulate this shift in response. Recognizing what stress feels like is the first step to shifting your response to stress.

What does stress feel like?

Stress is the body's way of telling you that it needs a break and it is extremely important to listen!

I have suffered from chronic stress twice in my life. Both episodes were related to unreasonably high personal demands (film production around the world while training for a world record attempt and working with my PhD project). As a result, two of my world record attempts failed (2002 and 2004) – and I usually do not fail to achieve my goals. Since then I have not had stress, and I have won all the World Championship competitions I have aimed for.

My symptoms of chronic stress were unmistakable: wandering eyes, incoherent thoughts, lack of focus, sleeplessness, loss of appetite, fatigue, despondency, a "pounding" heart for long periods of time during the day and night, abdominal pains, indigestion, night sweats etc. When you are stubborn like me and get that far, it is no longer healthy.

Fortunately, I came out ok on the other side of both incidences and know today what I should not expose myself to. I have become better at saying "no". Apart from the fact that the lesson cost me dearly, there is still a silver lining in that I am now in a position where I can empathize with others suffering from stress. When I give a lecture in a company and talk about stress management, I am happy to have experienced it in my own body and not just read about it in a book.

Control your stress!

Today stress has developed into a popular phenomenon and approximately one in four employees is expected to suffer from stress. It is hard to believe that it has come this far, and in many instances the stress may even be caused by the fact that these people believe they have stress, which in a manner of speaking is a kind of stress in itself. Stress from believing you are stressed has no real foundation and is really a misbelief about one's own ability and goals that are unrealistically high.

Two key elements in human nature separate us from animals: cognitive abilities (thoughts and conceptions about our existence and self-image) and the ability to consider the future and make plans for it. The second ability makes it possible for us to prepare ourselves for changes in the future, predictable as well as unpredictable. Unfortunately, it also gives us the ability to worry about future events – even events that will never occur. I believe it is a combination of our worries and the unpredictability of life that stresses us the most today rather than a great or unreasonable work load.

The attention which stress has received in the last decade has a both positive and negative value. The fact that stress is taken seriously is positive because it is not a coincidence that a Danish study revealed that headaches, migraines and sleep disorders have doubled within the last 20 years. The negative part is that you can suffer stress simply by thinking about it, whether a "danger" is eminent or not!

Since stress, as well as its underlying factors, are a natural and inevitable part of our lives, it is unavoidable. Our overall quality of life, physical health and even longevity depend on our ability to control stress. More and more courses in stress management are being offered to employees as well as to the unemployed. It has been shown that those who are unemployed are far more stressed than when they were previously assumed, because an identity crisis and a feeling of being inadequate are strong psychological stress factors.

I have not taken a stress management course myself, but I believe that the courses offered are very theoretical. I do not believe this is an effective approach because it is difficult to "think" away thoughts about stress. It is possible to use more thoughts to change your thoughts, but certainly complicated. I believe that a practical and pragmatic solution rooted in the physical act of conscious breathing will have a much greater effect. People who suffer from stress simply need concrete physical actions to change their mental condition.

I know of no better or more effective tool for change than your breath, combined with relaxation and meditation. As this book will reveal, these are crucial points in relation to mental control because they are easy and tangible methods to stimulate parts of the nervous system which mediate calmness. At the same time, those parts of the nervous system that cause stress are inhibited.

The following is a short list of suggestions for specific exercises, which you can perform to relieve your stress and enhance your well-being:

1. Daily relaxation – rest, meditation, imagery, slow and deep breaths, slow exhalation.
2. Exercise several times per week – walk, run, swim, etc.
3. Listen to music – soothing or joyful music, which bring good vibrations.
4. Laugh – because it stretches your diaphragm and lungs, & relieves tension in the solar plexus – a center of bad tension.
5. Do something you like. Take a walk in the woods, go fishing, enjoy an intimate moment, watch a good movie, visit your friends or write a letter.
6. Think positive – the glass is always half full.
7. Enjoy the fact that you are living, be grateful!

A couple of years ago another method to control stress was created in the US. It is a little device called a "StressEraser". This device works by simply putting your finger on a pulse sensor. On the attached monitor you can follow how your breathing should work to achieve an optimal state of relaxation in the body and brain. The device not only measures your pulse, but also very fine details in the working heart, called Heart Rate Variability (HRV). HRV reflects the beat-to-beat alterations in heart rate.

The HRV phenomenon was discovered in Russia and is quite new to modern science. However, in yoga, it is quite basic. In particular, the part of yoga termed pranayama has a focus on controlling the breath.

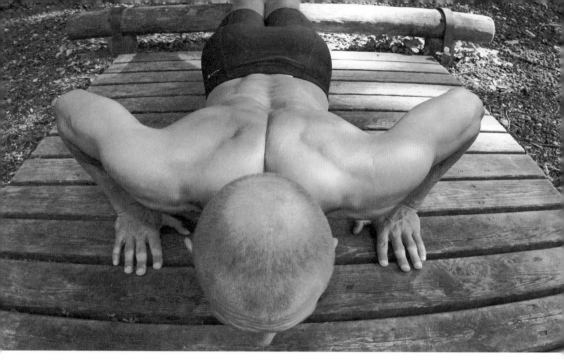

Physical activity is excellent against mental stress.

Ideally, you should try to adjust your breathing so that your inhalation as well as your exhalation follow a four heartbeat rhythm. This pace is very relaxing. In one fundamental pranayama exercise, you double the time of your exhalation (8 heart beats). This slower pace for breathing has an enormously calming effect on your nervous system. This exercise also reduces the hyperactive parts of your nervous system that are characteristic of stress. Your tolerance to stress is thereby increased both on a physical and mental level.

"StressEraser" is a good and well thought out product, and offers an excellent example of a useful tool which emerged from the fusion of thousand-year-old Eastern philosophy and modern technology.

I am in no way sceptical towards this device, but as a freediver I am used to a more simple and practical approach and thus tend to avoid complex technical instruments. The link between your breath and your heartbeat is undoubtedly more practical – and it gives you a greater sense of your body.

Another excellent way to manage stress is to hold your breath. Given the correct instruction, the so-called *diving reflex* is stimulated. As a result, the soothing part of the nervous system is also stimulated. It is the body's "relaxation-switch". I use breath holding in stress management for the same reason – both on myself and on participants in my courses.

Recent scientific studies have actually shown that when you are submerged in water and practice breath holding, many "alpha waves" appear in the brain, demonstrating a completely calm and relaxed state of mind – a form of meditation or trance. Alpha waves are also linked to a comfortable and timeless state of mind. This state is called *flow* in sports psychology – which is extremely favorable to achievement – particularly when under stress.

> "Because of a lot of pressure at work, I hadn't slept a whole night for months. After Stig gave a presentation on breathing and stress management and guided all the employees into the water for breath holding at our "kick-off" arrangement in the company, I slept like a baby all night long. The breathing exercises have helped me immensely, and I use them on a daily basis."
>
> Jakob Christiansen, 33 years
> Sales manager, CityMail Denmark A/S

In summary, breathing and breath holding act as a link between your body condition and state of mind – helping you control stress. As mentioned previously, stress can also be managed by gaining control of your thoughts. In many instances this can be more difficult than breathing exercises, since it is restricted to the brain. Let us take a look at a few simple techniques which can supplement breathing exercises.

Thought control

In the spring of 2006, I qualified as a freediving instructor at the Apnea Academy under the living legend Umberto Pelizzari. At the course, a sports psychologist said something that really stuck with me: "Your mind is very clever" – the more you think about this utterance, the more sense it makes! Your mind is phenomenally clever, and if you can learn techniques that link your subconscious mind to your consciousness, you can do the most incredible things.

> "Imagination is more important than knowledge."
> ALBERT EINSTEIN

Thought control is very effective because it works from the inside out. A controlled thought dictates the body's reaction, and thus, is a good starting point. As mentioned earlier, the breath is the perfect tool for controlling your restless mind, but with training you can also use certain thoughts to control other thoughts. In sports psychology, different "thought techniques" are adopted to suppress or replace negative or unwanted thoughts. Below is an example that you can work through to try it out.

Suppose I say the only thing you may not think about now is a polar bear - the only thing in the world that you may not imagine is a big, soft, white polar bear with a wet nose! Easy? Not quite. The simple task that you were given was not to think about a polar bear. But in doing so, the only thing you could think about was the polar bear! You will soon learn how to make the polar bear disappear.

Our thoughts and our mind are an inconceivable jumble of colors and forms. But it is difficult, if not impossible, to have more than one thought at a time. The single thoughts can be so tightly linked that they seem to flow together – this is how our line of thoughts works. If you hold on to one single thought, it is called concentration, and a single thought can only be held for a couple of milliseconds! When you continue focusing on one thought for several seconds, you enter a state of meditation. Practice this before you go to sleep – try stretching your last thought before you drop off to sleep. It is not easy.

But let us return to the polar bear that you were not allowed to think about or imagine. Now think of a long-legged giraffe. A big and beautiful long-legged giraffe on a dry savannah in Africa. Close the book for a moment and imagine this majestic giraffe. Close the book NOW. What happened? Did you see a beautiful giraffe? Yes – well good. Did you also see a polar bear? No, you did not, did you? – Excellent. Your thoughts dissolved the polar bear all by themselves and were replaced by something else. In this way you can easily control your thoughts and use positive thoughts to replace negative ones.

However, a current trend within the third wave of cognitive therapy steers away from the act of trying to control or actively change our thoughts. *Acceptance and Commitment Therapy* (ACT) aims at observing the thoughts without getting entangled in them. Thoughts can be treacherous and misleading and are not necessarily truths. A negative thought is dissolved by simply observing and accepting the thought passively. You might have heard of *mindfulness* which perceives thoughts as leaves floating down a stream. Mindfulness exercises are also a part of ACT.

If I get the feeling that a negative or unwanted thought is entering my mind during a dive (e.g. a polar bear!), I immediately replace it with a different thought to hold on to – it could be a giraffe, but I use other images. In the same way you can form such "key thoughts" or images that you can utilize, when your mind becomes stressed. When you dissolve the "stress of your mind", the undesirable effects on your body also disappear. If you link these thoughts to a steady breathing, it will work even better. We will be taking a closer look at this in the chapters on powerful breathing and soothing breathing.

The polar bear/giraffe example may seem banal, but the technique works brilliantly, especially if you practice it. In this kind of thought control you utilize a very strong capacity in your brain, namely imagery.

Imagery and visualization

When the subconscious mind accepts your conscious images, they become a part of your reality.

> "I use my breathing exercises, when I have to "warm up" my lungs. It makes me feel fresh and prepared for the training of the day. I also use them when I prepare mentally (visualizing my race). Before a race, I use them to raise my pulse, or if I need to calm my nerves."

> Jakob Carstensen, 31
Three-time Olympic games participant and
World Champion in 400 meters freestyle

When you think in images, you use certain areas in the brain which can create a global view of a situation and consider it in its full. Thinking in images or patterns enables you to understand contexts or situations in a split second. This is why symbols are so powerful. If road signs consisted of long sentences, it would not be easy to move safely through traffic.

In modern times, we predominantly utilize our analytical and logical brain capacities and are not very trained in using the intuitive and spatial parts. Consequently, there often exists a culturally determined imbalance in the brain. Luckily, through visualization you can create greater harmony.

When you think in images, you create a state that inhibits stress and promotes relaxation. This is why you must use your imagination, and this is why I believe in dreamers and visionaries.

"If you can dream it, you can do it"

WALT DISNEY

It is said that "faith can move mountains" – this proverb wasn't just made up.

Our thoughts are a result of infinitely fast processes in the world's most advanced and complex system, namely your brain. It is commonly accepted and recognized that "psychosomatic" sufferings exist; meaning that instability or an overtaxing of the psyche manifests itself as one or more illnesses in the *soma*, the Greek word for "body". As you have read in this chapter, it is actually this mechanism that lies behind stress. Within a few years the greatest threat to health in modern society is predicted to be stress and the complications it entails. Oddly enough, the opposite reasoning is less accepted. The logical perception that the psychosomatic phenomena can be turned into a positive, relieving, strengthening or even healing direction is less common. Many (because of ignorance or for illogical reasons) associate this notion with healers, superstition, magic, witchcraft, voodoo or something else. This is a shame, but fortunately a change in attitude is occurring these days.

In the field of psychology, a movement called "positive psychology" has emerged. It is concerned with looking ahead and using individuals´ potential and resources from the human psyche. Research shows that the brain cannot distinguish between something which actually happened in the physical world and something that just occurred in your mind. In other words, the brain is able to "cheat" itself, and to a great extent, you can push this illusion in a desirable direction. For example, physically injured athletes use thought exercises to be able to return to their sport just as "sharp" as before. Furthermore, a US study found that children who used thought exercises and visualization became better at shooting baskets than a control group that did not use thought exercises.

A Danish author and storyteller, Johannes Møllehave, writes down five things that have made him happy during the day before he goes to bed. This is an excellent idea for several reasons. First, the last thoughts you have before you sleep largely determine the quality of your sleep. Restlessness and negative thoughts result in poor sleep, while positive thoughts encourage a calm and balanced sleep.

Second, thinking about positive experiences has a beneficial long term effect on the brain, because positive "thought tracks" are laid down in your brain cells. A positive influence of the psyche stimulates the secretion of the "happy hormones", *dopamine* and serotonin, which strengthen the brain and simply provide us with feelings of well-being and satisfaction. At the same time, the production of the stress hormone cortisol is inhibited, helping the brain to remain sharp and bright. Collectively, the overall stress level decreases, affecting your health in a positive manner. Thus, thought exercises and meditation have been proven to lower blood pressure, pulse, regulate blood sugar (thereby being good news for type 2 diabetics), reduce asthma symptoms, depression and fear, to mention but a few examples. The small positive vibrations you yourself create in your brain can affect your cells and their functions – a transformation at the molecular level, which leads to a true metamorphosis of your body and soul!

> "Our life is what our thoughts make it"
> MARCUS AURELIUS

The more you believe in the power of thought, and the more you listen to your breath, the greater changes you can create in your life. This is why prayer works for so many people. In my yoga prayer, I am grateful for the good health of my family, my friends and myself. I am also thankful for life, and to those who suffer or experience hardship in the world, I send out positive and strengthening energy. Naturally, the energy waves I send out into the world will reach out and do good in some way or another. Forgiveness also lies in prayer and by forgiving people, negative thoughts leave your brain – the polar bear disappears!

A thousand years of wisdom and positive vibrations are contained in the word Amen and in the Eastern mantra *Om* (*Aum* - the symbol above). By saying them out loud or just thinking about them, the chemistry of your brain and the great fountain of your hormones will immediately change. Your brain becomes a better place to be, and stress disappears.

With the power of thought, we can accomplish miracles – if we believe in them! Let us join together and make the proverb "you become what you think" just as obvious and natural as "you become what you eat". It is just a matter of will!

(Un)health in modern society

Even though conditions are favorable for an ideal life in the prosperity of modern society, something must be going wrong because we are living ourselves to death. It is a tragic-comic paradox. The World Health Organization (WHO) of the United Nations estimates that roughly 40% of all the illnesses and "premature" deaths in the Western world today are related to our lifestyle. "Bad habits", such as a poor diet, smoking, alcohol, and lack of exercise are the primary causes. Worse, the current prognosis is that this figure is expected to increase to 70% in 2020 – a very gloomy perspective. In particular, recent increases in heart and vascular related diseases, certain forms of cancer, type 2 diabetes, dementia, depression and brittleness of the bones will be responsible for this pronounced rise.

The good news is that there is a bright light at the end of the tunnel. A British study has shown that you can add 14 years to your life if you quit smoking, restrict your alcohol consumption, eat healthy, fresh and diverse foods and exercise a little every day. All it takes is a change in lifestyle and commitment combined with the ability to take responsibility for your own life as well as your children's lives.

Statistics and analyses can mislead, but I believe that in relation to the British study, these estimates seem very reasonable - especially when I look at my beloved grandmothers. They drink alcohol in moderation, eat healthy food, don't smoke and all-in-all have an iron constitution. My paternal grandmother, Asta, who daily takes her dog for a long walk around the meadows, is 92 and takes care of her garden and farm on her own. My maternal grandmother, Stina, does morning gymnastics (with push-ups) and practices water aerobics, she is 96. I hope and believe that my grandmothers will live to their 100 year birthdays, especially because they are both mentally fresh and function well.

In addition, I believe that their strong health is due to good mental health including their cheerfulness, gratefulness and satisfaction. Recent studies have shown that not only exercise, but also an enriched environment, stimulates the formation of connections between new nerve cells in the brain, which can prevent various degenerative nervous disorders like Alzheimer's disease and dementia.

What can we do with stress?

There is no doubt that stress creates costs for individuals as well as industry and health care systems. In some instances, workplaces provide employees with the possibility of exercising and some even offer stress management courses, but do they suffice?

An easy place to start is the body because it is so tangible. Focusing on physical strength and well-being when it comes to nourishing employees, is narrow minded in many ways. Just as it is bad policy in medicine to treat only symptoms rather than focusing on prevention or problem-solving, it is also problematic not to include emotional and psychological aspects of health.

Exercise is undoubtedly healthy and will promote mental as well as physical health, but there are limitations to solely muscular work and fitness training. It can only do so much, whereas with the proper mental tools, you can perform quantum leaps.

For the same reason, teaching efficient breathing and a different mental approach to challenges are two of the basic elements of my company, BlueConsult, and my concept of breatheology. The challenge is now to promote the message and the techniques as fast as possible. In collaboration with Bjarne Brynk Jensen, who works with business development, I am developing and distributing this new approach to health. Bjarne is a company coach, a consultant for the Winter Olympics in Vancouver in 2010 and not only has broad experience with international organizations, but also has personal experience with work related stress and excess weight. We have created a concept where we introduce the point that a physical as well as a mental fitness rating will become a future competitive parameter for employees and business strategy. From this, we will work with self-development directed towards both top managers and employees.

We aim at developing harmonious people who, through an enhanced emotional intelligence, are willing to take responsibility for themselves and their employees by linking professional management guidance and cognitive techniques (from elite sports and positive psychology) with breathing exercises (from yoga and freediving). Since people use only 50-60% of their breathing capacity, a huge unexploited potential lies in breathing and will be given particular focus. If we are able to teach people to utilize just 10-20% more of their lung capacity, the extra energy could lead to a more productive working day, better decision making, greater well-being and naturally, fewer sick days. We believe that the concept has a future, but this holistic approach may be a couple of years ahead of its time.

In every part of society, a healthy and long-sought change in the attitude towards nutrition and diet is taking place. At work, fruit and organic food items are being offered and a more nutritional diet is now on the agenda. Our diet plays an important role in our well-being, so this change is positive and needed - probably also more than what people believe.

Diet

The food we eat is often regarded as just fuel for the body. Energy is delivered to the engine and the system stays running. But the type of food we eat and its quality also play a crucial role in determining our mental condition. This is the reason why yoga highly recommends unprocessed vegetarian food. The more prana (life force) food contains, the more active you will become on a physical as well as mental level.

Try during the day to become aware of how your body and mind react to what you eat. If you want to learn more on this subject, I suggest you study *ayurveda* – a classic Indian science concerned with health and herbal medicine.

Your breath is also closely tied to your food intake. The decomposition of food and energy uptake already begins in the mouth, and when your breath is calm and deep your digestion is stimulated by the soft massage of your diaphragm. Your visceral organs will secrete the appropriate amounts of digestive fluids and hormones, and more blood will pass around your intestines to absorb the decomposed nutrients. The more you can activate the part of the nervous system that calms and promotes digestion, the better you can utilize the energy in the food you have eaten. Since your breath is closely tied to your mental condition, you will have a greater urge to eat healthy food in active periods with plenty of fresh air. Whereas, in periods in which your breathing is poor, you will tend to eat food with more sugar and fat – or possibly not eat at all.

Fattening times

If we take a quick glance at the "obesity-statistics", the picture that emerges is terrifying. It is food for thought that we live in a part of the world where we are dying from overeating, especially when you consider that thousands of people each day on earth die from starvation. It is a tragic and unfair imbalance that needs to be changed.

In the United States, 60% of the population is overweight. As a teenager I lived in Florida and have visited the country on several occasions thereafter. Each time I am surprised to see a noticeable increase in obesity as well as how obese we humans can become. The last "case" I am familiar with was a young man weighing almost 1000 pounds. I encourage you to watch Morgan Spurlock´s movie "Super Size Me" - it is scary!

The problems of overweight people and obesity are much tabooed, and the fact that I use the word "obese" in this book may provoke indignation. However, if you do not speak openly about this problem and do not create practical solutions, you are doing people, especially children, a terrible disservice. It must be in the interest of all, both on a human and an economic level, to create a better and healthier life for individuals that suffer from obesity.

Fortunately, awareness of a proper diet is increasing – not a second too soon. Also, attempts to offer healthy eating options are being made in institutions and schools. Scientific studies using mice as well as children show that a healthy diet sharpens concentration and enhances motivation - thus multiplying learning ability and memory.

Being healthy with regards to food does not have to be difficult. Whether you wish to maintain your weight, lose weight or perhaps gain weight, I present a magical formula here.

A health treatment – the magical formula

Energy is often calculated in calories that are defined as the amount of energy needed to increase the temperature of one gram of water by one degree at an atmospheric pressure of one. The word calorie originates from the Latin *Calor* which means "heat". Sometimes the unit joule (J), which corresponds to approximately ¼ calorie, is used. The prefix "k", which reads "kilo" denotes a thousand as in kcal (a thousand calories) and kJ (a thousand Joules). To muddle things further, the designation "cal" is sometimes used instead of kcal. Thus it can be quite a challenge to keep up with your calorie intake if you are forced to perform long calculations constantly. It does not become easier when people often say calories but actually mean kcal!

In reality, it is quite simple:

$$E_{intake} - E_{consumption} = 0$$

E_{intake} is your daily intake of energy.

$E_{consumption}$ is your daily energy consumption.

The incredible feature of this formula is that you can easily forget about diets, pills and slimming powder from various clinics and magazines – you do not even have to count calories, weigh your food or calculate your daily energy consumption. All you have to do is eat nutritionally sensible food that is healthy and varied. In addition, weigh yourself every day or week. If your weight increases you have three options: a) eat less, b) do more exercise or c) both. Said in another and more direct way: If you eat too much you become too fat; if you eat too little, you become too thin.

It is very important that you listen to your body and know how you feel in your everyday life. Direct your attention to how various foods affect you. You know that French fries soaked in oil or soft drinks with sugar are fattening, but you may not consider the fact that they also can make you lazy, reduce your ability to concentrate, make you moody and altogether give you a heavy and sluggish body.

However, if you eat a lot of vegetables, fiber rich bread, chicken and fish and drink a lot of water, you will quickly experience the difference and feel more balanced. You will have more energy, be more active, feel lighter and your brain will work better.

It is no great surprise that several scientific studies have showed that you become more intelligent, happier and are able to concentrate better when you eat healthy foods and exercise – it is common sense.

The acid-base balance in the body

It is extremely important that your body is in balance. Let me be more specific with what I mean by this. To maintain a healthy lifestyle, it is necessary to achieve stability - also known as homeostasis.

Life depends on maintaining the environment in each living cell within certain parameters. A good example of this is our body temperature and the acidity of our blood, which should be maintained around a pH value of 7.4. Our breathing is crucial to this balance. By varying our breath under different circumstances, the concentration of carbon dioxide

(CO2) and thus the amount of hydrogen ions (H^+), which determines the blood pH, can be regulated. If breathing alone cannot maintain stability, the kidney is able to take up or release H^+ and thereby re-establish the balance.

It is not the blood alone that has to maintain a certain pH balance. It is also crucial for the rest of the body's tissue and bones. This pH or "acid-base" balance is, to a great extent, dictated by the food you consume. Within modern medicine this topic has achieved very little attention, since the emphasis in nutrition is on the energy in protein, fat and carbohydrates (kcal). However, the positive effect of base-forming foods such as vegetables, fruits and nuts is receiving more attention. In contrast, sugar, fat and protein are acid-forming.

Almost 100 years ago a Swedish doctor, Ragnar Berg, was the first to discover the connection between the acid-and base-forming properties in our food and our health. His rule of thumb was that we should eat 7 times more vegetables, potatoes and fruits each day than other types of food. Professor Olav Lindahl continued his work, which successfully applied base-forming foods to relieve pain for patients with arthritis, sciatic nerve pain and back problems.

Briefly, the hypothesis states that acid forming foods, such as sugar and fat, leave behind acidic compounds when they are decomposed in the body. This accumulates over time, leading to a weaker immune response. Thus, diseases can more easily attack the body. In contrast the base forming foods should neutralize the negative side effects of acids, thus providing a strengthening and curative effect. The issue is very controversial, but if you search for information on "alkaline diet/food", you will notice that the issue is a "hot potato."

I have been able to confirm positive changes in my body in periods where I have consumed large amounts of broccoli, grape fruit and nuts (for instance up to my recent world record attempts). I believe that most vegetarians will be able to report a more "light" and supple body. One of the reasons that yoga renounces meat is not only due to the idea of karma, but also that large amounts of meat stiffen the body. Two world record holders in deep diving, William Trubridge from New Zealand and Natalia Avseenko from Russia, are both quite fanatical about alkaline food and believe that the effects include: muscle strength, improved stamina, optimized oxygen consumption, and a delayed formation of lactic acid allowing for a shorter recovery time after hard training.

Try to aim at an optimal balance consisting of 75-80% base-forming foods and 20-25% acid-forming foods. This will also work as a sensational slimming diet that in a healthy and natural way restores the balance

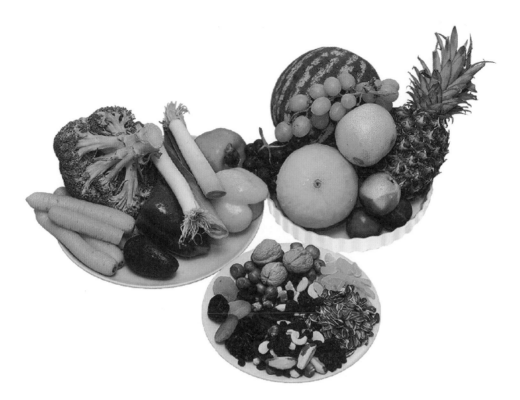

Citrus fruits, dark vegetables and nuts provide the body with valuble antioxidants, vitamins and minerals.

in the relation between fat and protein. At the same time, the body is emptied of accumulated fluid that is bound to acid residues in the tissue.

Why not embark on a little "scientific experiment" on your own body? Try living healthy for a week. Cut down on sugar and saturated fatty acids. Apart from the fact that you most certainly will feel more comfortable, you will also come to realize the amounts of unhealthy foods you chow down. One can of soda contains about 10 teaspoons of sugar – try adding up from there. Everything in moderation, so find your own balance – your body's perfect homeostasis. Below follows some ideas for your new diet.

Dietary tips

Breathe slowly when you eat. Breathe through your nose, chew slowly and repeatedly on every side to crush the food, absorb as much as possible through the mucous membranes in your mouth, secrete more saliva to enhance digestion and the absorption of nutrients from the intestines into the blood. Eat slowly so you can enjoy and taste the food!

It is a very common mistake to think that in order to lose weight or be in good shape you have to stay away from fat. Your brain and most of the nervous system are made of fat. Furthermore, fat is also a part of the cell membrane, acts to form a number of hormones, is important to the body's metabolism, etc. A good example is the fatty substance called cholesterol, which many believe is evil and only bad for you. In fact, your liver actually produces cholesterol because you need it. The cholesterol content in your blood is determined by what you eat, how much you exercise, your genes, etc. Two types of cholesterol exist – LDL (Low Density Lipoprotein) which we are taught to believe can cause hardening of the arteries, and the positive HDL (High Density Lipoprotein) that is said to have a protective effect on your vascular system. However, I encourage you to read the exciting and ground-breaking book "The Cholesterol Myths" by Uffe Ravnskov, MD, PhD. If you read it, you might be surprised! If you eat "Mediterranean food" and lead an active life, you will be able to affect your cholesterol number positively. Below follows some advice on a better lifestyle:

> Cut down on coffee, tea, soda, cakes and fat food. Forget about manufactured food products and pre-cooked food items. In doing this you avoid heavy metals, hormone residues, additives, artificial sweetening etc.

> Eat plenty of fruits and vegetables, particularly dark green ones, because they contain a good deal of nitrate, which aids the energy process of the cells. Garlic is also good for the lungs as well as the rest of your cardiovascular system.

> Eat legumes, nuts, seeds, red berries, grape fruit and dark grapes. These are all base-forming and full of minerals and vitamins.

> Remember to eat enough fat, but of the right kind: omega-3 fatty acids, olive oil, avocado, etc.

> Drink plenty of liquid – when your fluid balance drops by just 2%, your endurance capacity decreases by about 10%. However, do not consume large amounts of water every day, since it washes out salts from your body.

> Eat a big breakfast, carbohydrates for lunch and a supper rich in proteins. Good protein sources are fish, light meat and tofu. Green lentils, beans and chickpeas are good vegetarian protein sources.

> Eat a variety of foods and never too much at a time. If you want to exercise wait at least one hour after a big meal to enable the body to digest the food. If you are planning to do strenuous exercise, two or three hours are necessary to allow the blood to absorb nutrients from the gut and to leave the gut again. After you have eaten you can easily go for a quiet swim without drowning or getting into trouble.

> Dark chocolate (containing as high a percentage of cocoa as possible) has a good antioxidant effect and contains many healthy components. The same holds true for red wine, which contains iron and in moderate amounts also decreases the detrimental effect of LDL-cholesterol and increases the beneficial HDL-cholesterol.

> Also try "super foods" like the algae *Spirulina* and *Chlorella*, which are said to be the most complete source of nutrients, and make sure you get plenty of minerals like calcium, magnesium and potassium.

> Eat plenty of vitamins – especially vitamin A, C, E and the trace elements selenium, manganese and zinc, which all have an antioxidant effect.

Antioxidants and free radicals are often spoken about, but you almost never hear about how and why they work. I will briefly explain it here. Free radicals are atoms and molecules that have lost one of their paired electrons in the outer shell. Thus, they are highly reactive and eager to steal an electron from the first atom they encounter. In other words, free radicals change the configuration of other atoms and molecules destroying them in the process. Antioxidants have the ability to neutralize free radicals by donating electrons. In essence, it is wise to eat plenty of antioxidants to avoid aging and natural wear and tear of your cells. This keeps you healthy and resistant to various diseases.

Here are two recipes for raw food shakes – and apart from being base-forming they are full of antioxidants, good vitamins and minerals:

Magic potion 1
1 avocado
1 cucumber
1 lime or lemon
1-2 handfuls of fresh spinach leafs
½-1 cup of tofu
Soy milk
Liquidize – add ice cubes if desired

Magic potion 2
½ potato
1 beetroot
1 stalk celery
2 carrots
3 pieces of broccoli with stalk
4 radishes
Liquidize – add ice cubes if desired

If you follow the dietary advice above, your body, as well as your breathing, will become more smooth and efficient, and you will achieve considerable surplus energy. By cutting down on acid-forming foods with sugar, fat and protein, you reduce the oxygen consuming elements in your body. These not only contain small amounts of oxygen but also require more oxygen to burn. More oxygen can dissolve in an alkaline environment than an acidic environment. Thus, you gain a number of advantages by changing the chemistry of your body.

By now, you should have acquired a better sense of the importance of your daily food intake for your health and general well being. The old proverb you were taught as a child still applies: "You are what you eat".

Unfortunately, there are no easy solutions to the huge problems related to poor diet, smoking, alcohol and lack of exercise in society. Natural ways to start making a difference include: developing greater self-insight, focusing more on happiness, nurturing consideration for oneself and others, shifting to a healthier diet and increasing your physical activity. We just have to get going.

If you are willing to think out-of-the-box, a (pro)active approach to breathing could be a good suggestion. Especially in connection with weight loss, the right breathing could be worth its weight in gold. Breathing exercises can be used as a fabulous slimming formula.

Sympathetic slimming formula through breathing

I would like to add a little story about my friend Umesh who is 34 years old and holds a PhD in atomic and molecular physics. Umesh is a dedicated scientist, and the mission of his life seems to be an infinite focus on natural science. He is actually one of the most scientific scientists I know. The point of mentioning Umesh's educational background is to emphasize that Umesh does not believe in just anything. But, he believes in good breathing and has benefitted from it.

A couple of years ago he had a problem with his weight. Earlier in his life this had never been an issue, but years of sedentary work in the laboratory, combined with an unhealthy diet and varying mealtimes, had left its mark on Umesh. He got sick more often and had a feeling of being out of balance. In addition, the weight condition strained his back and he developed back pain. This made it difficult for him to walk far. He also suffered chronic sinusitis which lead to intense migraine attacks with a throbbing pulse in his temples at least once a month. The fact that he was born with the cartilage in his nose blocking the air passage through the right nostril made matters even worse.

While he was living in India, he participated in a course on pranayama (breath control) with exercises aimed at losing weight. There were no physical exercises like yoga positions, running or weight lifting in the course. The duration of the course was seven days and most exercises were performed while sitting. The breathing exercises included steady alternate breathing through the right and left nostril and also more powerful inhalations and exhalations. These were conducted with certain positions of the hands -so called "hand locks". There were largely no restrictions to what the participants were allowed to eat; however, the participants were asked to refrain from drinking coffee, tea, soda, alcohol and very fatty or heavily spiced food. The exercises were performed twice a day and each session lasted about 35-40 minutes.

On the second day, his appetite disappeared and he did not even feel hungry. Umesh continued with the exercises after the course and ate normally. The exercises were to be followed for 40 days in a row. If you forgot a session you should start over again on a new 40-day period.

Umesh lost 12 kg (26 pounds) after 14 days. Since then, more kilos followed and subsequently his weight has been normal and stable. Since the course, he performs 30 minutes of breathing exercises each morning on a daily basis. Apart from the weight loss, his right nostril has opened and he no longer suffers headaches or inflammation of the sinuses.

Just as hibernating bears and other hibernating mammals may lower their resting metabolism and can do without food for an entire winter, the human body may also markedly increase its metabolism – especially when most of our billions of cells acquire optimal conditions and work together in a well-balanced, synchronous system. This is exactly what happens when you adopt the correct breathing and mental exercises because the metabolism of your body, as well as the absorption and utilization of the food we consume is multiplied. This not only occurs when performing the various exercises, but continues for hours because the nervous system and the organs of the body are vitalized and boosted.

By now you have covered quite a few pages and your brain has been working hard, so now it is time for you to activate your body and invite it to join the game. Let us proceed to the practical exercises.

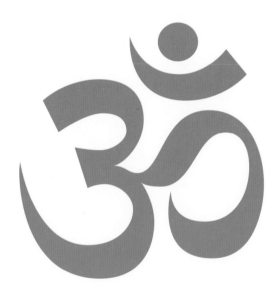

"We learn to do something by doing it.
There is no other way."

JOHN HOLT

Exercises

Relaxation, concentration and imagery

Fortunately, the art of relaxation is easy to master. The challenge is to remember to do it in a busy and chaotic everyday life. Discovering peaceful moments in which you can take a mental or physical break can change your life immeasurably. If an imbalance exists between your body and your thoughts, neither will function optimally. Combining relaxation, concentration and imagery can help you move towards balance and an optimally functioning body and mind.

One reason anyone can learn to relax and achieve greater focus is that we are all breathing beings. Your breath is always with you, and apart from keeping you alive, it is also the best tool you will ever have to adjust your body and your thoughts. By consciously grasping your physical breath, you can influence your mental processes. When you make your breathing deeper and slower, your thoughts will automatically follow. Therefore, breathe as softly and calmly as possible during these exercises. After a couple of weeks or even a couple of days, you will increase your capacity to relax and concentrate at will, and you can harvest the fruits of you efforts.

An objective of mindfulness and ACT is to get in contact with the present moment, in order to accomplish full awareness to your here-and-now experience and to become open and receptive to what you are doing. With an attentive breathing you will achieve a here-and-now experience because it provides you with a physical anchor point that is connected to your nervous system and mental state.

If you find it challenging to relax and concentrate in the beginning of your training, it is perfectly okay. Often it takes a while for the body and the mind to slow down. Focus on your breathing and let is flow as naturally as possible. Once your body and mind have calmed down it is much easier to concentrate on the specific task at hand.

The amazing part of using this kind of "brain gymnastics" is that the technique is widely applicable and can be used in any possible connection – at work, in the bus, before a meeting or prior to an athletic feat etc. When you master the technique perfectly, a few seconds will be enough for you to relax and concentrate. In other words you will be able to take a "power rest" that is more effective than any powernap!

Are you aware of your senses?

We perceive the outer world through our five senses. Spend some time reflecting on what type of perceiver you are! Are you the more visually oriented type, who remembers things that you have seen more easily, or are you more of an auditory person who remembers things that you have heard? Think about which favorite relaxing past time activity you indulge in – do you listen to music, do you visit a museum or do you prefer to be physically active? By tuning in on the senses you spontaneously use every day for relaxation, you also create a greater consciousness about the senses that you can activate in your relaxation exercises. The obvious way to become more insightful into your nature is to train and intensify the awareness of all your senses, but begin with the sense that is most natural to you.

Create a peaceful environment

Tranquillity and stillness are extremely important, when you have to "listen" to your body and work with your mind. In time you will learn to relax and concentrate even in a noisy and stressful environment, but start in a peaceful place with the exercises. Make sure that you have plenty of time and create your own "space" where you can work with yourself and your breathing. Take off your watch, turn off your cell phone and prepare yourself for a pleasurable activity. If you are very busy, you can either postpone the exercises or just do one or two of them. Do not hurry through four or five exercises just because you want to get them done. It is anything but productive!

The best position in the World

When you are going to practice relaxation and concentration, lying on your back is perfect. The Earth's gravity pulls equally on your body which means that the fluids in your body such as blood and lymph do not have to move against or with gravity. This physical balance at once reduces the body's metabolism because the muscles, and especially the heart, do not have to work as much and thus peace is mediated to your mind.

Do not lie on something too soft, but use for instance a blanket, a yoga mat or a camping foam mat. The spine has to be relatively straight and follow the floor. If you are very sway-backed, it is helpful to place a little pillow or a rolled up towel under your loin. This may also be necessary with your neck, but remember that it needs to be aligned with your natural posture so that you do not create tension in either your neck or throat. Possibly try pointing your chin slightly down towards your chest. You can also lie on your bed or on the couch – it is up to you to decide whether the surface is hard enough!

When you lie on your back in the *Relaxed Position*, make yourself as slack as possible. Spread your legs a little and let your feet drop to the sides. Likewise position your arms slightly from the body with the palms of your hands turned upwards and fingers slightly bent. Close your eyes, but make sure that you do not fall asleep. However, if you are very tired, go to sleep and postpone the exercises.

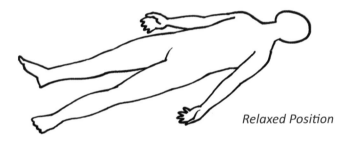

Relaxed Position

When you have finished practicing, you should return slowly to the "real world". Wriggle your toes and feet a bit, move your fingers and slowly open your eyes, when you are ready to do so. After that carefully roll to your right side and slowly sit up. Rest and smile for a moment before you stand up.

You can easily do the exercises on your own, but it may be beneficial to do them with a partner who can read the exercises aloud (in a calm and pleasant tone) until you are familiar with them.

The exercises below can help you in your work with relaxation, concentration and visualization. As described, exercises may work differently from person to person, so find the exercises that work the best for you.

Five exercises for relaxation, greater body awareness and imagery

1) *GRAVITATIONAL FORCE*

Notice how your entire body feels heavy and relaxed. Focus on all the points of contact with the material below you. Your heels, calves, the back of your thighs, buttocks, back, shoulders, forearms, elbows and the back of your head. Notice how your completely relaxed tongue lies in the bottom of your mouth. With a little bit of practice you will be able to sense the skin "sliding to the ground" particularly around your eyes and cheeks. When you become able to release all the tension in your muscles and thoughts and let gravity work on your body, your visceral organs may also feel heavy and relaxed. The word "heavy" does not refer to an unpleasant or a heavy pressure, but to a soft and comfortable pressure or pull.

2) *SOUND PICTURE*

Try forming a picture from the sounds that surround you. Listen carefully and you will discover that your ears are capable of hearing sounds that you would not notice in your everyday life. Think about how blind and weak-sighted people have a more finely tuned sense of hearing, making it possible for them to hear when they walk past a tree or an open door. You can also train your ability to hear in this exercise, and you should try to picture as many images as possible. Take your time. If you hear a bird sing then imagine the bird's colors, its shape, size, where it is sitting and so on. If you hear voices then try to imagine what the people look like, how they are dressed, how many there are etc. The more alive your images become, the more you train your hearing and your ability to visualize. Try to move through the entire sound spectrum and listen to details and words without dwelling on them for too long or relating to their meaning. Listen to the sounds as a "mumble" from which you can create your images.

3) *BLUE-RED BODY*

Imagine that your entire body is blue. Completely blue. Now try to imagine that you are changing color. The blue now, gradually and controlled, changes to a deep, clear red color accompanied by a pleasant warm feeling. Begin with your toes and move slowly up your body – ankles, shin, knees, thighs, hips, loins, stomach, back, chest, shoulders, arms, hands, and finally the neck and head. Be particularly thorough with the lower jaw, tongue, cheeks, eyes, forehead and the top of your head. Feel how the crown relaxes, add a little smile to your lips, and feel how the part of the body you focus on becomes warmer.

4) *ECSTATIC JOY*

Try to remember a very important and emotional event in your life – perhaps a fantastic sports triumph, a final exam or some other great goal that had a special significance to you. It can also be an intense experience like the birth of your first child or a watershed experience in your childhood. It goes without saying that it must be a positive and powerful experience that makes you happy and relaxed. Try to relive the moment as clearly as possible – what was your feeling? Where was your feeling located? Also try to make it clear why this incident made you so happy! The more you practice evoking this feeling, the faster you can do it in situations where it can be of help to you. Thereby you can create your own effective "relaxation remedy".

5) *PARADISE*

Imagine a beautiful and serene landscape. It might be a magnificent mountain, a forest lake, green, wavy hills or a sunlit ocean. You can also travel back to a place you were fond of in your childhood - for instance the back garden of your parent's house or at your grandparents or perhaps a pleasant "secret" place. Try to sense all the different smells the place you are imagining had – the long grass with morning dew, the many colorful flowers, the freshness of the clean air in your nostrils, feel the temperature, humidity etc. Likewise imagine all the sounds – trickling water, chirping birds, buzzing insects, wind blowing leaves etc. In time you will be able to train your mind to such an extent that you can enter your own paradise at any time and any place.

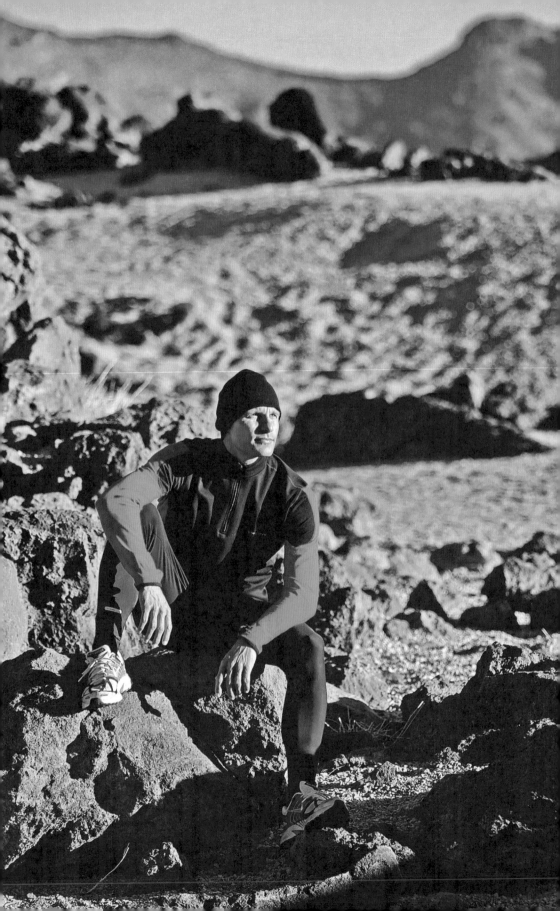

Normal breathing

Good and bad habits

Why do we breathe?

People breathe in very different ways, but how you do it is not unimportant! The purpose of breathing is to gain oxygen (O_2) from the air and to remove carbon dioxide (CO_2) from the body. The more you can control this process, the stronger your health will become.

When you breathe and air enters your lungs, oxygen is delivered via your blood, to every cell in your body. Here, oxygen is consumed in the *Krebs cycle* (citric acid cycle), which is a cascade of chemical reactions involving the transformation of the food you have eaten to energy-rich molecules called *ATP* (the cell's battery) by means of water and enzymes. The more effectively you breathe, the more energy you will be able to store in your body.

A byproduct of this cycle is carbon dioxide which blood transports to the lungs where it is released back into the air upon exhalation. If your breathing is sloppy and untrained, you will not be able to cleanse your body properly, which may lead to fatigue or headaches and affect your visceral organs negatively.

Plants utilize carbon dioxide and release oxygen using solar energy in a process called photosynthesis. Plants and animals thus depend on each other and live together in symbiosis.

Just as your body breathes, so "breathes" every cell in your body. Each cell can be viewed as an independent organism, since it produces its own energy and has its own cleaning mechanisms. In Indian yoga tradition, cells are referred to as "little lives" and your breath is so fine that is works on this level.

For you to stay healthy and well, it is essential that your cells are given the opportunity to maintain a good balance. An important component of this balance is to breathe properly.

Inhalation and exhalation

Breathing is composed of two parts – inhalation and exhalation – and with the appropriate method of breathing, an optimal balance between the two is achieved. This does not necessarily mean that inhalation and exhalation should take the same amount of time, but that equal amounts of air should be exchanged. If you exhale very slowly, your body will accumulate carbon dioxide. This kind of breathing is termed *hypoventilation* (*hypo* meaning "under" or "less than normal" in Greek) and causes headaches and other unpleasantnesses, which naturally is undesirable. Conversely, if you exhale quickly or forcefully, the body will suddenly lose much carbon dioxide leading to dizziness and a prickly sensation in your fingers and lips. This state is termed *hyperventilation* (*hyper* meaning "above" or "too much"), and can be experienced by nervous or stressed individuals. Of course, this is not a good way of breathing either.

Most people are not aware of the fact that they are breathing in an ineffective way. However, it is easy to learn how to improve your breathing. When it comes down to it, the aim is to inhale the same amount of air that you exhale. By strengthening and making the muscles of your rib cage more flexible, a more natural and harmonious breath can be achieved.

Inhalation begins with the outer muscles of the ribs contracting, making the ribs move out and upwards, which increases the volume of the rib cage. This leads to a lower pressure in the lungs, which through two membranes are in direct contact with the rib cage.

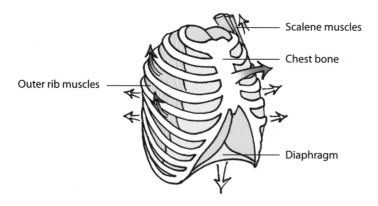

During inhalation the rib cage expands and the diphragm is lowered.

The greatest increase in volume is caused by the diaphragm. Its dome-shaped roof contracts and moves down towards the abdominal cavity drawing air into the lungs like a large piston. Because this movement is a result of muscle contractions, it acquires energy and is thus called an active process.

During intense inhalation or respiratory distress, an additional set of muscles around the rib cage and in the throat, particularly the large diagonal muscles and the scalene muscles, are activated.

In contrast, as a result of the elasticity that the lungs, thoracic cavity and diaphragm have achieved during inhalation, a normal exhalation is completely passive. The outer muscles of the rib cage relax and so does the diaphragm, which slides back into its natural curved position. This causes an increase in pressure in the lungs and the air to be exhaled.

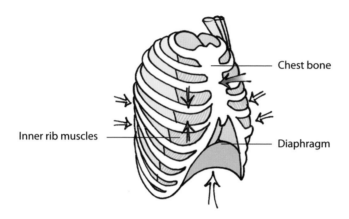

During exhalation the rib cage collapses and the diaphragm returns to its initial position.

If you are nervous or stressed, a bad habit can arise where your exhalation is performed actively. In this case you use energy on both exhalation and inhalation and create an unnatural tension in your body which in time will spread to your psyche. A relaxed breathing, with a completely passive collapse of the chest and diaphragm, is a very good habit to form, especially when you are busy with your everyday doings.

You may want to try breathing in different ways yourself, and with your hands, feel where and when the muscles contract and relax.

The large dome-shaped diaphragm is the pivot of the breathing process, and consists of a set of muscles and tendons, which in a relaxed state is convex and situated like an arch up in to the chest cavity. If you hold your hands around your body below your rib cage, you can feel how a large inner plate moves towards your navel, when you take a deep breath. This is the diaphragm. The name stems from the Greek word *diaphrassein* which means to separate or to be between. In the upper part of your body the diaphragm separates the chest cavity, which contains your heart and lungs from the abdominal cavity and its organs such as the liver, spleen and stomach.

In the front, the diaphragm is attached to the breastbone, on the sides it is attached to the lower ribs, and at the back to the spinal column. It is penetrated only by the esophagus and larger blood vessels. The diaphragm can be viewed as a large inner piston that can change the pressure of the chest cavity, as well as the abdominal cavity, and thereby influence all the organs in these areas. Not only does the diaphragm afford a steady and even breathing, but it also has an enormous influence on blood and lymph circulation in the body, which has not been thoroughly investigated yet. In our everyday lives, the diaphragm functions in coughing, throwing up, or when we go to the bathroom. This is also where the cause for hiccups lies, which is a row of involuntary contractions of the muscles in the diaphragm.

The most important function of the diaphragm, however, remains to be the ventilation of the lungs. Nonetheless, only a few use it optimally, and many are thus cheated of the physical benefits a correct usage can provide. But with only a few daily exercises you can become best friends with your diaphragm.

Air's voyage into the body

If you want to be able to control your diaphragm and make it flexible and strong, it is extremely important to regulate the flow of air during your inhalation and exhalation. In order to train your breathing, it is important to understand how the respiratory passages and lungs function. Let us take a closer look at the passage that air takes through our body and what occurs during this passage. If you close your eyes and take a couple of deep breaths, try to feel the air flow in your body. Where does air enter, where does it flow to, and how does it feel? There are two entry points for air: Air can enter through the nose or through the mouth.

Let me make it clear from the beginning, the mouth is for food and should only be used for breathing when the nose is clogged or when working hard. There are many good reasons for breathing through your nose including the fact that your blood is better oxygenated in the lungs.

When air enters your nose, the many small hairs in your nose immediately filter out larger particles. Air then proceeds to the nasal *conchae* where it is humidified and warmed, and at the same time, smaller particles are filtered out by the surrounding mucous membranes. Indeed if we use our nose properly, we will be able to appreciate this extremely sensitive organ. The entire nasal cavity receives nerve fibers from the nervous system, and thus directly influences our health and state of mind. In the upper part of the nose there is a number of delicate sensory cells that can detect various smells and odors, and the information from these are directed via nerve fibers to the brain.

In spite of its impressive sensory function, the nose does not receive much attention either culturally or medically in the Western world. This could be rooted in the fact that in our age, where information has to be fast and accessible, visual communication is preferred. In addition, as "civilized" human beings, we have left our original nature behind, and do not run around "sniffing" each other – perhaps because it is not vital for the survival of our species!

However, unconsciously our nose is constantly in use and receives a wealth of information from our environment. We all know how odors can have an overwhelming effect on us, for example it may lead us back to a childhood experience or, if the smell is atrocious, make your stomach turn inside out. Primitive people use their nose much more and also dilate their nostrils more frequently than we tend to. Notice for instance how you smell a flower or perfume. You most probably dilate your nostrils and draw air up high into the nose.

As late as in 2004, the scientists Richard Axel and Linda Buck received a Nobel Prize for their discovery of an unknown group of odorant receptors on the olfactory receptor cells, their function and connection to the brain. This was a step towards a better understanding of how odors are intercepted and conceived. Nonetheless, there is still a great deal that we do not know about the nose. There is even an ongoing debate as to whether a sixth sense is present in humans – the so-called *Jacobson's organ*.

By breathing through our nose, we not only clean and warm the air, but also detect a plethora of important information from our environment. If you breathe through your mouth, this information is lost.

Deep down into the lungs

When air leaves the nose, it continues past the hindmost parts of the oral cavity's roof where the *uvula* is. Further down in the throat it passes the *epiglottis*, which is a little flap of cartilage tissue behind the tongue. If you are in doubt where your epiglottis is, try swallowing while feeling your throat. Also try breathing at the same time – is it possible? When you breathe, the epiglottis stands in an upright position, but it closes the entrance to your *trachea* to protect the lungs as soon as you swallow. In this way solid food and liquid is passed to the stomach without entering our trachea and lungs.

Not many people realize that without air we would not be able to speak, shout or sing. The *larynx*, which is our "voicebox" is situated immediately below the epiglottis. It consists of two vocal chords and various cartilaginous parts. When the vocal chords are pulled together and air is passed from the lungs, they vibrate and produce sound. It is an impressive precision of mechanics at work when the vocal cords produce this wealth of various sounds in speech or in song. The area between the vocal cords is called the *glottis*, and when it is completely closed, air cannot pass to or from the lungs. Accordingly, the vocal chords not only function in sound production but can also protect the lungs by closing.

En route to the lungs, air flows down through the trachea, which branches at the bottom to form an upturned Y. Air flows through the two thick branches called *bronchi* to the left and right lung. The lungs look like two conical sponge-like sacs that almost fill up the chest cavity. The largest is the right lung and is subdivided in to three lobes. The left lung consists of two lobes and has a cardiac impression to give room for the heart. Many imagine that the lungs are simply two bags that can shrink and expand. The lungs are in fact exceptional and beautifully branched structures reminiscent of large unruly corals.

The bronchi further divide into smaller branches (*bronchioles*) that are situated within the lungs. From here air finally reaches its destination, the alveoli, which are small air sacs resembling small grape-like clusters. It is in these small air sacs that blood and air exchange oxygen and carbon dioxide, and the alveoli are extremely specialized to perform this particular task.

Firstly, the cell wall of the alveoli is very thin in some places, merely a few layers of cells corresponding to less than a thousandth of a millimeter. Oxygen moves freely to the many small blood vessels (capillaries) that surround each alveolus. This is also true for carbon dioxide which moves in the opposite direction – from the blood stream to the alveoli. In addition, oxygen is dissolved in a soap-like liquid that covers the inside of the alveoli enhancing oxygen flow. This liquid also supports the alveolus so that it does not collapse when the lungs are emptied, and maintains that the alveolus is optimally dilated and in close contact with the blood stream.

The effectiveness of the alveoli is also due to there being so many of them. There are roughly 300 million alveoli which correspond to a surface area of about 150 m^2.

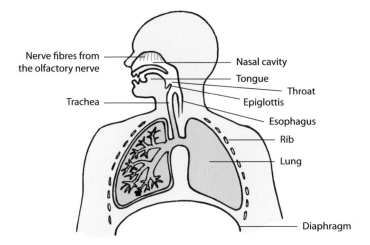

The upper airways and diaphragm.

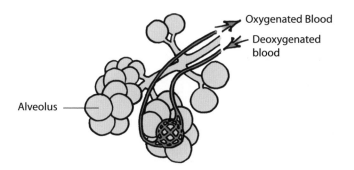

Deoxygenated blood from the body takes up oxygen in the fine capillaries that lie around the alveoli in the lungs.

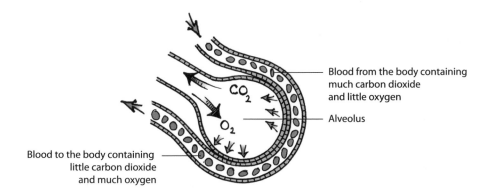

The distance between the capillary and the air in the alveolus is very short to allow carbon dioxide to diffuse into the alveolus and oxygen to be taken up by the bloodstream.

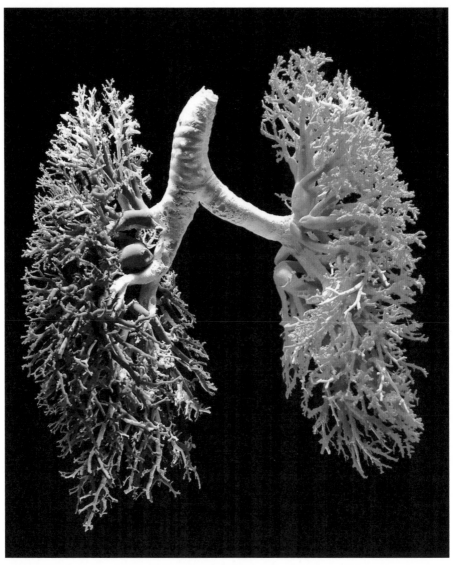

The human lung is extremely branched. Left lung (red) is smaller than right lung (blue) because the heart is positioned below the left lung. The red and blue color are plastic fillings for illustrative purposes.

Brain control of our breath

In the center of the brain lies a control tower which continuously makes sure that you breathe day and night. The nervous system automatically emits impulses to muscles in the diaphragm and chest, and at the same time receives signals when the lungs are full of air. This is the fundamental breathing that people take for granted because it is automatic. However, we may not consider the fact that in stressed situations nerve impulses restrict the breathing of the lung to half of its capacity. On the alveolar level this corresponds to a decrease in alveoli surface area to 75 m^2.

On the other hand, we have the ability to consciously change the rhythm and depth of our breath and thereby reestablish and even enhance the natural breath.

This ability to control our breath consciously is quite unique and differentiates us from other animals. For instance, the dolphin that in social behavior, size and intelligence resembles humans does not possess the ability to shut its consciousness and breathing down during sleep because it would simply drown. The dolphin has solved this problem by letting half of the brain sleep at a time.

Breathing is controlled centrally by the brain, where the brain

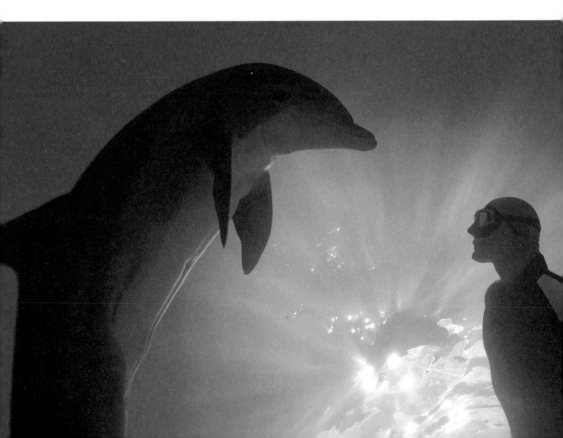

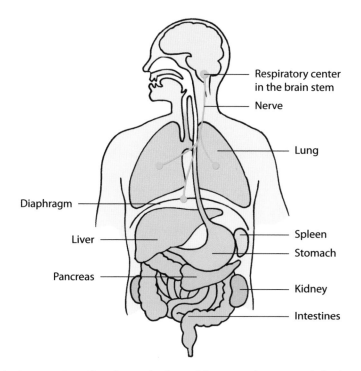

The respiratory center stimulates the breathing muscles around the lungs and in the diaphragm through a series of nerves (yellow).

stem that resides in the central and lower part of the brain regulates rhythm and intensity. It is usually an elevation in the amount of carbon dioxide and not oxygen, as many may believe, that plays the most important part in the regulation of our breathing. Small receptors in the brain stem record this elevation, and the brain accordingly emits signals to the muscles in the rib cage and diaphragm to increase their activity.

Next time you go for a run, perform an activity that elicits a rapid pulse or if you are stressed, try to end your session with a breath hold. You will promptly experience an intense urge to breathe, and this is not caused by lack of oxygen because your lungs are full, but rather it is caused by the fact that your body is producing carbon dioxide and is trying to get rid of it in a hurry.

When you have calmed down and gained a deep and slow breath, the diaphragm moves gently up and down rendering a comfortable massage to the visceral organs in the abdominal cavity.

In this way your liver, spleen, kidneys, stomach, pancreas and intestines are influenced, and with it your digestion, which promotes the secretion of various enzymes and hormones. By breathing efficiently, it is possible to elevate the pressure in the abdominal cavity and thereby intensify the massage of its organs, which has a stimulating, cleansing and slimming effect. This is another good reason for learning how to utilize your breath optimally by means of breathing exercises.

The living nervous system

The part of the nervous system that cannot be controlled by our will is called the autonomous nervous system. It consists of the *sympathetic* and the *parasympathetic* pathways that regulate the vital functions of the body. These can be influenced by inner and outer factors of both physical and mental origins. Both parts of the nervous system are continuously at work and do it in an antagonistic way to maintain a healthy balance.

The sympathetic nervous system is mainly activated by stress and prepares the body for a fight. In other words, it is a survival mechanism that increases heart rate, blood pressure, blood sugar and dilates the pupils. It is termed a *"fight or flight"* response. Evolutionarily, it is necessary to be able to react promptly when facing immediate danger, but if the sympathetic nervous system becomes overburdened by prolonged stress, mobbing or hard physical activity, it will wear on the organism and has the potential to lead to fatal consequences.

The parasympathetic nervous system, however, has a calming influence. It lowers the heart rate and blood pressure and simultaneously promotes digestion and the uptake of nutrients. It is termed *"rest and digest"*. Hence, it is primarily during rest, eating and sleeping that the parasympathetic nervous system dominates and coordinates the body's repose and regeneration. It is mainly this part of the nervous system that is advantageous to activate through breathing exercises.

Let us now consider one of the most fundamentally important elements in the parasympathetic nervous system, the *vagus nerve*, which is the most complex of all of our nerves. In Latin, *Vagus* means "wandering". It is termed so because from its origin in the brain stem it spreads nerve fibers to the throat and upper body, and through these nerve fibers signals wander to and fro between the body and the brain. In short, the vagus nerve connects the brain to everything from the tongue, pharynx, vocal chords, lungs, heart, stomach and intestines to different glands that produce enzymes and hormones, influencing digestion, metabolism, and much more.

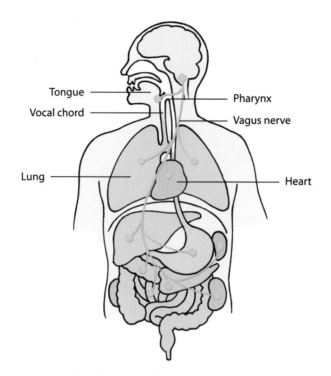

Tongue

Vocal chord

Lung

Pharynx

Vagus nerve

Heart

The large vagus nerve (yellow) runs from the brain stem down through the neck to lungs, heart and internal organs in the abdominal cavity and is a vital part of the soothing parasympathetic nervous system.

The vagus nerve's considerable influence on your lungs and heart and the connection to your brain is quite interesting. This trinity, brain-heart-lungs, rules your body and governs your mind. The key to managing your state of mind and stress level lies in being able to activate the calming parasympathetic pathways of your nervous system on command. Typically, the will cannot control this part of the nervous system, but if you hold your breath for a brief moment and then slowly exhale, the vagus nerve is stimulated bringing peace to your body and mind.

In effect, strengthening the living nervous system can pay off. And the best tool you can use is an efficient training of your breath. You can master this yourself. The path to this goes through training your breathing, which can be achieved by means of yoga.

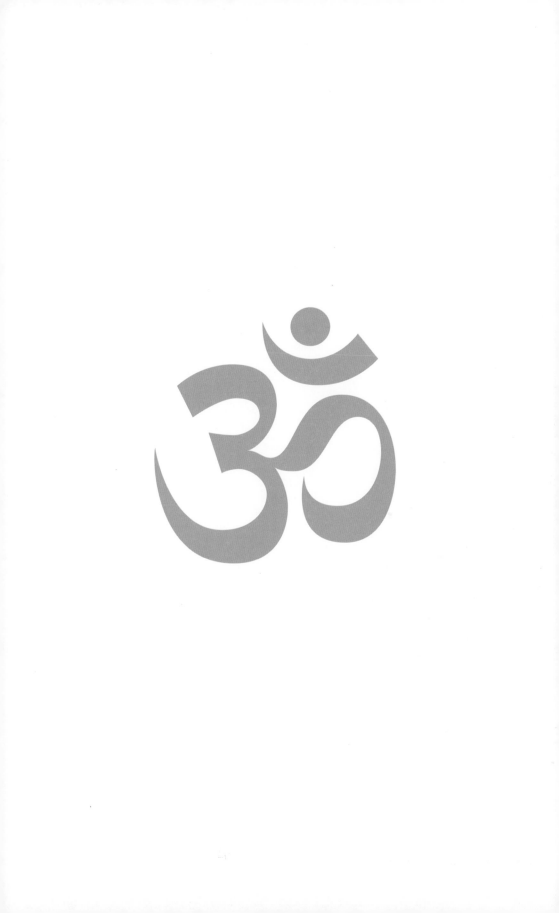

Exercises

As I have mentioned previously, relaxation is inextricably bound up with the parasympathetic part of your nervous system, the so called "rest and digest". It belongs to the self-propelled autonomous nervous system, but by actively focusing on your breath and the movements of your diaphragm, you can influence the system enormously through the vagus nerve that spreads from your brain to your lungs, heart and other organs.

In particular, when you exhale slowly or take a deeper breath than usual, the vagus nerve is activated. Try closing your eyes, taking one or two deep breaths and exhaling slowly with an audible sound such as a deep satisfying sigh. This will dilate your lungs and the rest of the chest, and the vagus nerve will release a signal to the brain to relax. It is sure to make you feel more comfortable. It might even have made you drowsy or sleepy, and if you did not yawn before, you probably will now. A large, lovely and lazy yawn! Notice how the lower part of your lungs and the side of the neck are activated when you yawn. It is pure electroshock on the vagus nerve – positively speaking!

If you think that the connection between your breath and mind sounds very plain, even banal, you are entirely right. At the same time it is certain that this connection is immensely overlooked and thus rarely exploited. It is a shame, so let us do something about it instantly. If you are still yawning, take four fast and powerful breaths – it is sure to stimulate you.

The next couple of relaxation exercises can be performed under the same conditions as the five exercises from the last chapter – that is lying on your back in a peaceful place. The exercises are similar to the previous exercises, but focus more on your heart, body and breath.

1) FEEL YOUR HEART

Feel your heart – in your throat, by your ears, temples, solar plexus, in all of the fingers etc. Imagine that you lower your heart rate (pulse) by using your mind – it can actually be done!

2) *BEAUTIFUL SELF-IMAGE*

Try looking at yourself from the outside or from above. Observe how harmoniously your chest moves slowly up and down. Observe how peaceful and relaxed you look, and particularly note how gentle and composed your breathing is. If your breathing seems a bit brisk or strained, then take a little time to reach a more relaxed breathing, so that in the end it seems elegant, effective and effortless. Consider filming yourself while you are breathing. Besides obtaining a strong and concrete image of your breath, it is quite motivating and satisfying to be able to monitor your development and improvements over time.

There are plenty of advanced and more extensive techniques by which you can improve your mental control and aid you in deep relaxation, concentration and ultimately meditation. You can research these exercises yourself, when you are ready for them. You can find out more about these topics either in books or through people, who can provide you professional guidance and help. You may also develop and try out your own new exercises. It is always fun and interesting to move down new pathways, and in the end it does not matter which technique you choose, as long as it is efficient and works for you. Once you have learned to relax and achieve a greater consciousness in your body and mind, you possess the fundamental skills necessary to work meaningfully with your breath.

The natural breath

Breathing exercises can be performed anywhere at any time. You will not be disturbing others because people will most likely not notice that you are exercising and exploring. Through your breath you will quickly be able to get in contact with your body, slow it down and increase your ability to visualize. Most yoga and breathing exercises are best performed on an empty stomach, but light exercises can be performed after a meal. In fact, it can be quite nice to relax after a meal and oxygenate your body to improve digestion. However, your pulse will be higher and your body's natural metabolism will be elevated after a meal because the food has to be broken down and absorbed. This will not make a difference, since the essence of the exercises is to focus on being conscious of your breathing. So close your eyes, listen, feel and say hello to your own breath.

Ensuing are four exercises that by strengthening the consciousness of your breath is certain to make it more natural and harmonious. The exercises can be performed in the *Relaxed Position*.

Commence by reading through the exercises and performing them afterwards, or have a friend or partner read them aloud for you while you perform them simultaneously.

1) *NEUTRAL*

Breathe through your nose. If you feel like breathing through your mouth or perhaps just exhaling through your mouth, this is okay in this exercise. Breathing naturally without changing your rhythm by thinking too much is the most important.

2) *ATTENTION*

The next step is to observe and improve the understanding of your breath. Breathe as described above, but notice how it feels when the air enters and flows into the lungs. Does the air feel dry? How far up in your nose does the air go? Do the nose hairs move? How does the air feel in the throat – does it tickle in the throat or does it feel comforting? Close your eyes and listen to your breath – what does it sound like? Where do the sounds come from? Are the sounds different when you exhale and inhale? Is the air warmer, colder and moister, when you exhale? Does the air touch your upper lip? Try breathing through your mouth. Does it feel more natural? More relaxing or more stressing? Is it easier to control and maintain a soft and natural rhythm in your breathing by doing it through your nose or mouth? Which type of breath enters deeper into your "stomach"?

The main purpose of this exercise is to notice every little detail of your breath – the better you get to know your breath, the more you will be able to change and optimize it. The challenge in this task is to observe and sense all these things without affecting your natural rhythm. Do not become frustrated if you forget to breathe or if the rhythm of your breathing becomes broken because your breath will soon reestablish itself. After you have performed this exercise for a couple of days, you will be able to observe your breath for a longer period of time without consciously changing it, and you will discover that your rhythm has become more soft and dynamic.

3) *RHYTHM AND PULSE*

You have now reached a better understanding of your breath, so it is time to take a closer look at the relation between rhythm and pulse. Try to understand your own natural rhythm. For example, how many times do you breathe in a minute? If you find it too difficult to count and time your breaths simultaneously, then try filming yourself or solicit a friend's help.

If you have a watch that can monitor your pulse, it will be quite simple, if not then place a finger on the carotid artery where the jaw bone turns up towards the ear lobe. If necessary, you can lie on your side – it will then be easier to watch the alarm clock beside you. If you cannot locate your pulse with the finger, stay on your side and listen to the pillow. You might be able to hear your pulse instead. Also try to play with the depth of your breath. When you take deep breaths or breathe quickly you will soon notice that the pulse rises. Try sensing how the pulse is directly related to the inhalation and exhalation. When you breathe in, the pulse rises immediately, and during exhalation it is slowed. Try taking a deep inhalation and feel the pulse. Also try to exhale very slowly – your pulse might even fall below your natural resting pulse (beats per minute).

4) YOUR NATURAL RHYTHM

Now to determine your natural rhythm. Look at the breathing curve pattern. This shows the respiratory cycle with one cycle consisting of an inhalation and an exhalation. Now try to time your personal respiratory cycle by recording how long it takes for you to breathe in and out 10 times at the pace you are breathing now. Divide this by 10 and you have a measure for one respiratory cycle. If for instance your respiratory cycle takes 5 seconds, you are to the right of the curve, as indicated by the numbers, and you are in a relatively relaxed state. If on the other hand your respiratory cycle takes 1-2 seconds, you are perhaps stressed or have done a bit of physical exercise. This estimated value will be the natural rhythm of the day. In time you will attain a deeper, calmer, more gentle and dynamic breath, whereby you move further to the right on the curve. When it manifests itself as a permanent and natural part of your "new" breath, you will undoubtedly experience the many positive physical and mental advantages an efficient breath can bring. Possibly note your daily rhythm on your calendar, and enjoy the progress you experience during the following weeks and months, which you have achieved through a greater awareness and training of your breath. If you are ill or stressed, you will soon notice that you are positioned further to the left on the curve and have a more sloppy breath, which naturally is not optimal.

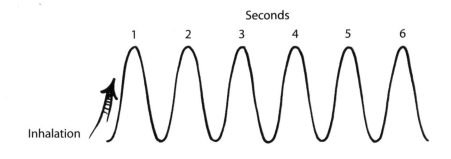

Breathing curve indicating seconds. If you are stressed, inhalation may only take one second - or shorter. If you are relaxed and calm, inhalation may take several seconds.

Part II

Conscious breathing

Part II will bring you through different aspects of conscious breathing. You will learn how to make your breathing more efficient and thereby create a stronger bridge between your body and mind.

Yoga will teach you how to become more aware of your senses and introduce the key elements in pranayama (breath control). You will also be introduced to the art of breath holding as practiced in freediving. Holding your breath may seem challenging but can be done safely and holds the potential to create a greater control of your mind. More focus on your breathing can also help you optimize your daily activities and peak performances in sports. Furthermore, using your body and breathing fully can give you a strong health. Should you fall ill, breathing exercises can also help you to recover faster. Finally, working actively with your breathing and your thoughts can soothe pain during illness, pregnancy and child birth.

The concept of breatheology is built up in such a way that your breathing habits will progress naturally when doing the exercises following each chapter. The various exercises will strengthen your breathing muscles and fine-tune your nervous system and help you reach your true potential.

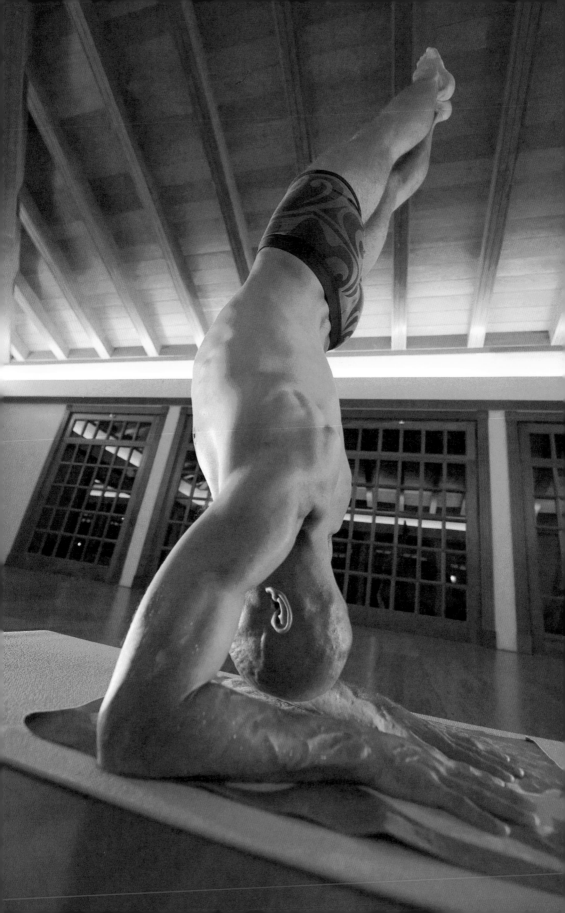

Trained breathing

Become healthy through yoga

Holistic outlook

Yoga is an ancient South Asian science and in our hectic Western world its justification is greater than ever. If you immediately associate it with nine tailed elephants, lotus flowers and sweet incense, worry not, it is not that odd at all: yoga has often been depicted as something mysterious and secretive.

In general the purpose of yoga is to provide you with a better life through greater self-insight into your body and thoughts. In yoga the breath is a central element because it can show you how to bridge the gap between the physical and mental you.

In the previous chapter you read about how your body is put together and how your breath works. This fundamental knowledge is extremely important, but even if you have read several textbooks on human anatomy and physiology, it will not improve your breathing. The second you combine your scientific knowledge of the body with practical breathing exercises, you will be able to profit fully from the time invested. Luckily, yoga is the proper pathway to follow, since no other discipline or science in the world is so detailed and profound with regards to the physical-mental connection.

In order to understand why the breath is so deeply rooted in the holistic world view that yoga starts from, it is essential to know the background and history of yoga. From this you can gather a more differentiated picture of the thoughts surrounding the relationship between body, mind and nature that through thousands of years have been passed on from generation to generation.

The great idea of yoga is that everything is connected and cannot be divided into isolated units. The word yoga originates from the root *yuj* which means "union". Yoga is a method to connect body and mind, mind and soul and the individual and the universal soul. Yoga is the reconnecting with your inner being and the merging with other people, nature and the universe. By expanding your consciousness it is possible to reach that which lies between your physical body and your existence, namely the soul. When the soul is liberated, it can establish contact with the universal soul of life. Viewing yoga in this way, you realize that yoga is much more than fascinating body positions, enlightening meditation and moderation. Yoga is the integration of love and ethics, offering a way in which you lead your life in this world.

Yoga is intended for the use of everybody, despite being originally created from a Hindu line of thought. In the old scriptures, yoga is described as *sarvabhauma*, which in Sanskrit means "for all". Thus yoga is created for all mankind and is possibly the world's oldest science and systematical method with the purpose of increasing health, preventing or curing diseases and establishing peace and happiness.

Yoga is merely one out of six classical systems that make up the core of thousands of years old Indian Hindu philosophy. According to this, the individual can develop and gain insight into the highest universal truth through yoga. It is obtained by rationally understanding the reality that the self experiences, as well as accepting and understanding the laws of nature and the forces that shape the universe.

The fundamental idea that the philosophical systems share is that the cause of all human suffering is an ignorance of our highest potential. Thus yoga is an art of life that prescribes how man, through discipline and knowledge, can cultivate body, mind and soul and thereby gain a balanced, healthy and happy life. Even though yoga starts from within the individual, the purpose is to benefit others as well. A healthy and harmonious human radiates positive energy and peace to its surroundings.

Yoga is not founded on a religious belief, but rather intended to be a starting point for a universal energy or soul that permeates and runs everything. The philosophy of yoga has spread to the larger parts of Asia and appears in various forms, such as Japanese Zen Buddhism and Chinese Taoism, and throughout history it has to some extent influenced the Western world. The most notable ambassador of yoga's humble and respectful philosophy today is undoubtedly Tenzin Gyatso, the 14th Dalai Lama of Tibet, who in 1989 was awarded the Nobel Peace Prize.

The pioneer of yoga is presumably *Pantanjali*, who wrote the classical work *Yoga Sutra* more than 2,000 years ago. Pantanjali did not invent yoga, but the Yoga Sutra is the oldest document that provides a theoretical, philosophical as well as a practical background for yoga activities.

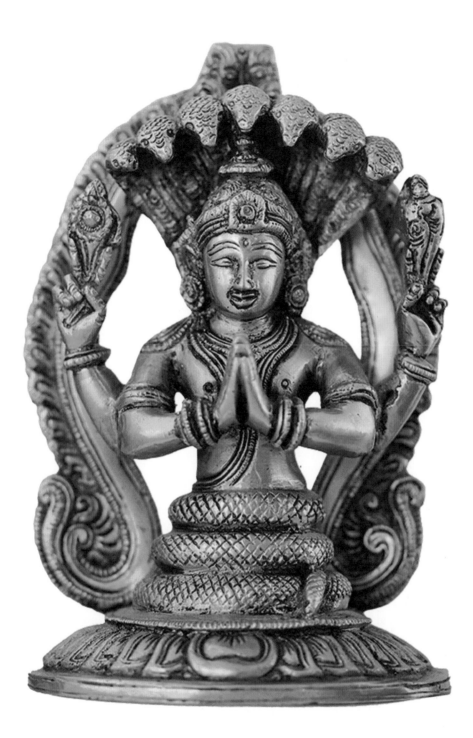

Pantanjali is believed to have written the first classical yoga scripture. Here he is presented with a seven-headed cobra curled around him.

Like many other practical disciplines, yoga cannot be intellectualized, but has to be exercised via experience. Best is to find a competent yoga teacher, who can teach yoga proficiently and show the positions and provide guidance in the principles of yoga. If such a teacher cannot be found, it is still interesting to broaden your knowledge on yoga and carefully try some of the basic techniques.

The advantages of yoga

The fruits of yoga are called *Siddhis*. They appear as changes in your body, mind and soul. In Sanskrit *Siddhi* means something that is achieved, completed or fulfilled. Some of these qualities are: a good appetite, digestion, a sweetish body smell, clean sweat, clear saliva, less mucus, absence of illnesses, high spirits, a strong psyche, good looks, a slender figure, glowing skin, clear eyes, beautiful voice, less need for sleep, great courage and enthusiasm, full strength and control of the sexual urge.

> "Yoga works on your conscience. Yoga works on your consciousness. Yoga works on your intelligence. Yoga works on your senses. Yoga works on your flesh. Yoga works on your organs of perception. Thus, it is known as the global art."
>
> B.K.S. IYENGAR

Anyone who practices yoga a couple of times each week can gain these advantages. If you practice intensively, the changes will be particularly distinct. In 2003 when I was training to break the freediving World Record for the first time, I was very disciplined and committed in my daily yoga performance. I experienced many of the changes mentioned above and had an enormous amount of energy. In addition I only slept five to six hours each night, but woke up completely restored and fresh each morning. It was a very positive period during my life, and I have no doubt whatsoever that it was caused by the many hours of practicing yoga and relaxation. Previously, in other periods of my life, I had been practicing sports just as much and equally as hard, but never before had I experienced such harmony and energy reserves.

We are aware of the fact that yoga positions, to a greater or lesser extent, influence the body by changing blood circulation, massaging the internal organs and hormone producing glands, and strengthening the nervous system. In effect, they are very useful in boosting daily health and are eminent tools when treating conditions like metabolic imbalances, elevated blood pressure, stress, diabetes, asthma, complications of the lungs, impure skin, indigestion, overweight and depression to name a few.

As well as clear-sightedness and clear-hearing, more supernatural results exist, such as the ability to enter another person's body, become invisible, have wishes granted, expand in space, control everything, repress lust, fly, reach wherever you wish to go (even the moon), and to live off of atoms. However, these siddhis are not only difficult to achieve, but are also difficult to understand and require knowledge and control that lie far beyond the attainability of most people.

But if you would like to know how to become invisible, I suggest you read about how light is deflected or how to camouflage. If you would like to know how to live off of atoms, I suggest you read about "sun gazing" or particle physics. If you would like to know how to enter another person's body, I suggest you study psychology. And if you would like to know how to fly, I suggest you fall in love!

The eight elements

Ashtanga is the basis of yoga. The word originates from Sanskrit and means "with eight limbs". In The Yoga Sutras, Pantanjali systematically describes the eight parts that comprise the complete yoga system and leads the practitioner (the yogi) to the true goal. *Buddha* lived almost contemporarily with Patanjali and there are many obvious convergences between yoga and the commodious and charitable Buddhism. In particular with respect to moral concepts, but also with regard to tolerance towards other religions, respect for living creatures and nature and an acceptance of human diversity.

The eight elements in ashtanga are as follows:

1) *YAMA* – GUIDELINES FOR GOOD BEHAVIOR IN SOCIETY

Non-violence and no harm (either in thought, speech or in deeds), truthfulness, freedom from possessiveness and greediness, control of sexual urge and unselfishness.

2) *NIYAMA* – GUIDELINES ON AN INDIVIDUAL LEVEL

Cleanliness (food, thoughts, body etc.), satisfaction, enthusiasm, extension of the intellect and belief in and a surrendering to God or the divine.

3) *ASANA*

Dynamic, steady, comfortable poses that cleanse, strengthen, stabilize, and make the body more supple.

4) *PRANAYAMA*

Breathing exercises that assist in cleansing the body and mind, so that life energy can move more freely.

5) *PRATYAHARA*

Controlling the senses – either by calming them to render them passive, or by leading them inwards (abstraction). The first stage of concentration of the mind.

6) *DHARANA*

Concentration or complete attention.

7) *DHYANA*

Meditation – concentration on a higher level. The mind focuses into one point or dissolves during a longer period of time.

8) *SAMADHI*

The final goal of yoga where body, mind and soul are freed, and converge into one point where they are united with the universal life energy. Often termed *Nirvana*.

The first two elements, yama and niyama, are a set of universal rules for positive human behavior that are independent of time and place. Living by these ethical guidelines result in a positive cleansing effect on an individual as well as cultural level. Furthermore, they are regarded as foundational and essential to moving forward in yoga.

Practical exercises compose the next level and consist of asana, pranayama and pratyahara. They mobilize and discipline the body and mind of the individual. In time they lead to the last level that is the inner and spiritual part of yoga consisting of dharana, dhyana and samadhi that together lead to a deeper understanding of life.

Different "schools" that lay down how yoga can or should be practiced have appeared throughout time. *Karma yoga* focuses on the actions or deeds of individuals, *jnana yoga* on knowledge and intellect and *bakti yoga* on devotion to the divine, just to mention a few. It is less important whether you devote yourself to this or that "school", because they are all connected and converge at the same point. Yoga is yoga, and the goal is always the same – to ease your mind, to gain control of your thoughts and actions, and in the end to unite with the universe and eternity.

From body to mind

The most prevalent type of yoga in the Western world is *hatha yoga*. Hatha yoga is characterized by the cleansing and empowering of body and mind through physical exercises starting from the breath. This physical dimension makes hatha yoga attractive as well as accessible, because it resembles something we have seen before – sport and training.

Traditionally hatha means "determined", "stubborn", "powerful or "effort", and this type of yoga leads to control of the will. The body is used as an instrument to subdue thoughts and to control the mind.

If only the physical aspects of hatha yoga are used, it is called *ghatastha yoga* (*ghata* means "physical effort"). Modern expressions like "fitness yoga" and "power yoga" that flourish within gym classes are within the same category, even if they do not derive from the original exercises' rhythm and succession. In many instances "power yoga" has a positive effect on physical health; but if there is no aim to ease the mind, to gain self-insight and control of your thoughts, and to experience the divine within you and within the universe, the deeper meaning of yoga and - possibly life - is lost.

On the other hand, it can be argued that the yoga styles that exclusively focus on a devotion to a God or knowledge (bhakti and jnana yoga) lack emphasis on the physical aspect. In the end it all comes down to finding a healthy balance.

As mentioned, it is important to understand that hatha yoga in its original form was not only based on physical aspects, even though the very bodily centered asanas (yoga postures) and pranayama make up the central parts. Like other kinds of yoga, hatha yoga is built on a moral foundation, and the aim is to reach the highest form of meditation and fusion with the universal energy.

The ultimate purpose is to gain complete bodily control, especially control of the breath, through strict discipline and the study of the scriptures over time. When the energy of life, prana, flows harmoniously and in complete balance between the two nostrils and the rest of the body, it is united with mind and soul in the divine. For prana to flow freely, it is necessary to cleanse the channels of energy (*nadis*), which directly correlate to the blood vessels, the lymphatic system, nerves, intestines, glands and spine.

Detox through yoga

I do not aim at presenting all the different cleansing methods here, but I will emphasize three that with a little practice can be successfully performed by all. The first method is nasal cleansing which consists of rinsing the nose and sinuses with lukewarm salt water. As mentioned previously, breathing through your nose has many advantages. The cleaner and more open it is, the more sensitive it is, and this is of particular value when you start performing the advanced breathing exercises.

The act of nasal cleansing or *neti*, as it is called in Sanskrit, is done by pouring the saline solution into your nose by means of a special container with a long spout. Cock your head to one side and pour the water into the uppermost nostril. When the nasal cavity is full, the water will run out of the bottom nostril, or it may run out of your mouth. Lukewarm salt water (equivalent solution to body water, approx. 0.9% salt) is usually used and can be made by adding roughly a teaspoon of salt to a jug of water (9 grams per liter).

Every experienced freediver or scuba diver is familiar with a similar technique for cleaning the nose and sinuses if they are blocked. You close one nostril and directly suck up sea water into the other nostril. Then you close both nostrils and lean your head backwards to allow the water to enter the sinuses. Apart from the obvious advantages of rinsing the mucous membranes of dust, bacteria, old mucus etc., a nasal cleansing also relieves breathing and improves your sense of smell and taste. In addition, the method is a good preventive measure for colds and can relieve or eliminate complications like nose bleedings, allergy and *sinusitis*. Nasal cleansing also has a protective effect on the lungs, because the mucus membranes will work properly and eliminate harmful microorganisms before they enter the lungs and develop into serious diseases like *pneumonia*, *bronchitis* or *tuberculosis*.

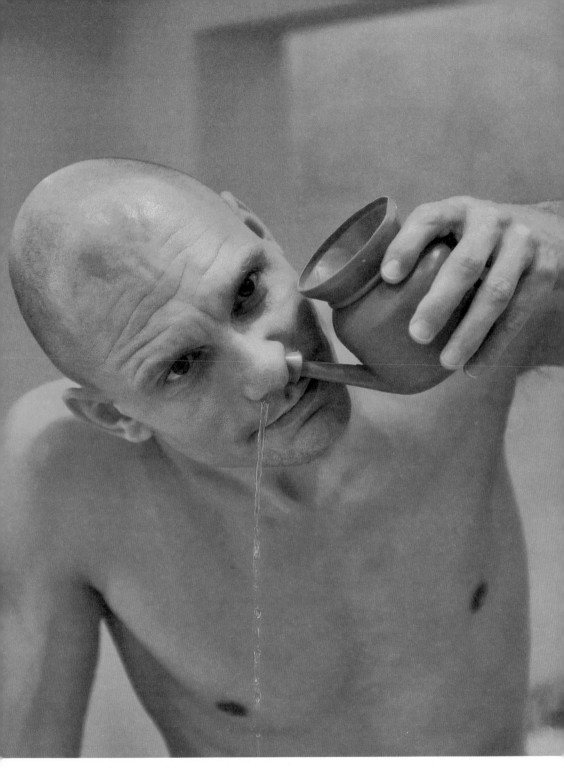

Warm salt water cleanses the nose and sinuses by removing dust and bacteria and improves breathing at the same time.

Another method that cleanses the nose, sinuses, blood and brain involves a simple breathing exercise. A series of powerful "puffs" through the nose is produced by activating the abdominal muscles and muscles of the diaphragm. Though the exhalations are active, the inhalations should be a passive, natural response. A third and highly effective method involves tightening, isolating and even rotating the abdominal muscles that twist and turn like a snake through the center of the abdomen. This process cleanses and stimulates the intestines, stomach, spleen, pancreas and all of the other organs in the abdominal cavity leading to an improved digestion and metabolism. However, this third method takes quite some practice and body control.

When your body has been cleansed, it has to be strengthened and shaped to be able to build up and retain energy (prana), whereby health, body-consciousness and vitality are automatically obtained. This is achieved through certain body positions (asanas) that constitute the third element of the yoga system, and is much more than merely body building. Each position has to be performed with complete control over each muscle, nerve fiber and thought. The advanced asanas may appear impressive and complicated or even painful. However, it only appears that way because each position has to be performed with effortless ease. Otherwise it is not yoga, but acrobatics or circus stunts. In other words it is important to progress slowly and not forcefully. I clearly remember what my Indian friend Umesh once said during a yoga session: "Yoga is evolution, not revolution" – it is very true.

Every yoga position is designed specifically to access and benefit organs, e.g. the lungs, liver, brain, glands etc. When the body is consciously manipulated in this way, each cell works optimally. You should not feel tired or weakened afterwards, so relax and concentrate at the same time when you practice yoga. Take deep and harmonious breaths and remember to put a little smile on your lips. The final goal is to be able to sit motionless for longer periods of time during the breathing exercises, concentration and meditation, because a motionless body allows the mind to calm down. Spare a minute now to take a couple of slow and deep breaths – preferably with your eyes closed. Does it not mediate calmness and well-being?

Composure of the senses and mind

The breath provides an easy access to gaining insight into the body and mind, and since it unites the two, breathing is essential to all yoga exercises. Let us turn to pranayama or breath control, which is the type of yoga that forms the basis of this book.

> "For he, who has gained control over his breath,
> shall also gain control over the activities of the mind.
> The reverse is also true. For he, whose mind is in control,
> also controls the breath. The mind masters the senses,
> and the breath masters the mind."
>
> HATHA YOGA PRADIPIKA

With pranayama you achieve a higher energy level in your everyday life, and you are granted the opportunity to reach a greater sense of self-insight and self-control. The word pranayama can be translated in several ways. Originally prana refers to "the energy of life", but also covers concepts like the breath, wind, life, vitality, energy and strength. Ayama can be translated as regulation, expansion or dimension. Pranayama is often directly translated as "breath control". This is not incorrect, but the essence of pranayama is the ability to take up and manage prana mainly by using your breath.

The core of pranayama is to calm the senses and the mind by means of the breath, especially by working towards achieving a balance of the flow of air between the two nostrils. In fact, almost every other hour the balance between your nostrils shifts. Close one nostril at a time and breathe in - which nostril dominates right now?

In the human mind an endless stream of thoughts constantly swell up from the subconscious, and sense impressions in particular will shape and control our thoughts. Perhaps the expression "flood of thoughts" is more pertinent, because the active brain runs in top gear. Asian Indians talk about "a monkey mind", because our thoughts are forever jumping back and forth like a little monkey. New ideas constantly emerge like fireworks in a clear night sky. The art is to be able to orchestrate this firework display, so that all the rockets are fired at once – or completely subside. For instance, if you are very stressed or terrified, it is difficult to tell yourself, "relax, everything is under control", because your thoughts are swirling around consciously and unconsciously. However, you will always be able to take hold of your breath – it is easy and very practical.

An old Tibetan proverb states: "The breath is the horse, the mind is the rider", and it is this intimate relationship between the horse and rider you have to think of when you breathe. If the horse is annoyed or unbalanced, it will fight against the reins, and the rider will be jerked from side to side. Likewise, an angry and inconsiderate rider will experience problems with the horse if pushing it around, because the horse is stronger than its rider. However, when horse and rider are in harmony, they will merge and become one as well as help and support each other. That is breath control – and it is just this that we are about to tackle.

> "Through the last couple of days I have been reminded of the great benefits that relaxation and yoga contain, benefits that can be applied to all the facts of life, and which can make you a better sportsman, businessman, colleague, man, father and human. It sounds great, but if we forget to unwind daily from the rapid pace and stress of reality, we will never reach our full potential. To be able to provide top performances, you have to find the balance between strain and restoration. We are usually good at straining ourselves, but we often forget to relax and recover. We have to learn how we can enter a restful space and accumulate more energy before the next wave hits us."
>
> Ole Stougaard, 35
> European Team Champion Triathlon and owner of Multicoach.dk

More energy in life

As previously described, pranayama is the fourth element in ashtanga yoga, and basically consists of a set of breathing exercises that contain three parts:

> Inhalation (*puraka*)
> Breath holding (*kumbhaka*)
> Exhalation (*rechaka*)

The main objective is to take up and regulate the vital prana. Together with the fifth element, pratyahara, pranayama bridges the gap between, on the one hand, the "outer" yoga that is the moral and self-disciplinary aspects of yamas and niyamas (first and second elements) and the physical aspects of asanas (third element), and on the other hand the "inner" yoga that consists of the concentration and meditation found in

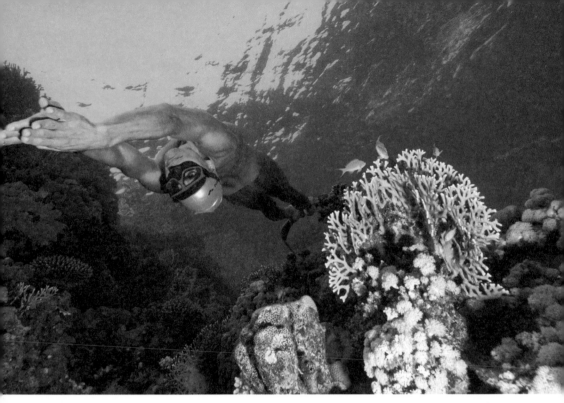

Breath holding in water is also a kind of pranayama and calms body and mind.

dharana and dhyana (sixth and seventh elements), ultimately leading to spiritual liberation or samadhi, the eighth element and the final goal of yoga. Therefore, in yoga it is in the connection of the physical world and body with the inner mind that pranayama and breathing play a central role.

It is not easy to define prana, but let me provide you with a couple of examples from everyday life. When you get up on a sunny morning with a clear blue sky, your energy level is likely to be higher than when you get up on a grey and wet morning. Let us presume that you have eaten exactly the same amount and type of food and performed the same work the two days prior. "Scientifically", your energy level should be the same. However, it does not feel like it. When you feel exuberantly happy and can feel powerful energy bubbling inside, it is prana that is neatly tied to your consciousness.

"Mind and prana are mixed like water and milk. Both of them are equal in their activities. Where there is pranic movement or activity there is mind (consciousness). Where there is consciousness there is prana."

HATHA YOGA PRADIPIKA

You have probably met people that seem to radiate energy that almost seem to have a shining "aura". Or perhaps you have felt how a person standing behind you was watching you – that energy and consciousness is also prana. If you have seen a dead animal or person, you will know that some form of energy is missing. Some call this energy the soul, and it is here that we are starting to conceive the meaning of the word. Prana is your energy, prana is your consciousness, prana is your soul. Any vibration in the Universe has its origin in prana's dynamic life energy – the driving force of everything. According to yoga and the Hindu line of thought, death occurs when the prana exits the body, whereby the force that drives our breath disappears. Likewise, it is prana that initiates our breath, when we are born.

The art of pranayama is to control prana in whatever shape it may take in the body. If prana does not flow freely, your energy level will drop and in the worst case illnesses will arise. Thus it is essential to maintain clean energy channels, or nadis, to let prana flow freely. Similarly, it is important to be aware of the areas of the body that can store or even block prana. These centers are called *chakras* and are key points in the energy balance of the body.

The energy system of the body

The word *chakra* means "wheel" or "rotating ring". The individual chakras are positioned where energy channels join in the body, and work as transformers that control the energies of the body.

The three most important energy channels are *ida*, *pingala* and *sushumna*. Ida starts from the left nostril and pingala from the right. They cross each other several times down along the spinal column which inner channel is called sushumna and is related to fire. Sushumna symbolizes the intense energy that can blaze up inside of you. Because different energies join in these centers, they can function as accumulators. If the system is out of balance, energy can be blocked in the chakras, and it is important to try to avoid this by cleaning the energy channels and to take care of the body and mind through breath control.

A set of chakras exists that are typically depicted as having different colors, symbols or elements, and each of these plays a certain role in the energy system of the body. Often seven chakras are described. It has been proposed that the chakras oscillate with different frequencies and thus emit light in different colors, and that sages of ancient India could sense and describe these oscillations. If you have not been working with

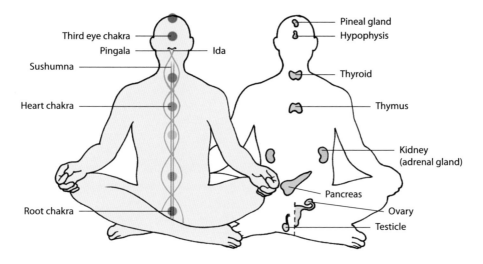

The left figure shows the seven chakras and energy channels. The important hormonal glands of the body are shown on the right.

yoga and the line of thought that lies behind it, the thought of such structures residing in the body may seem abstract and even superstitious.

The positions of the seven chakras do in fact coincide with important glands, nerve centers and blood vessels known to modern anatomy. However, it is crucial to emphasize that the chakras are not identical to these organs but rather intimately linked to them. The lowest chakra, commonly known as the *"root chakra"*, is positioned at the base of the spine between the sexual organs and the anus. In modern anatomy, this area is called *Os sacrum*, the holy bone. It is important to notice that exactly at this point the lower branch of the parasympathetic nervous system leaves the spine and contacts the sexual organ, digestive system etc. Seen from a psychological point of view, this chakra is related to the most primitive instincts: survival, sexual energy and fear.

The central chakra is the "heart chakra" that accumulates positive and cheerful energy from prana during inhalation. In our culture the heart as ever is the ultimate symbol of love. Today we are aware of the fact that the heart not only functions as a pump but also produces hormones, and considering the close relation it has to the brain through the nervous system, it is quite natural to ascribe the traditional qualities such as joy, wisdom and soul to the heart. When the heart beats gently we feel that we are well. This also holds true for our breath and our thoughts. When our breathing is calm and restrained, the mind relaxes. It is this trinity of heart, brain and breath that you must bear in mind, since it is the source of your well-being and health. The Roman physician, Claudius Galen, was aware of this and was the first to describe the pulse as an indicator of a person's health.

In the head is the "third eye" chakra, which is located between the two brows. It is active during concentration and meditation. The holy mantra Om is closely attached to this chakra. The Sanskrit term *ajna* means "command", and it is positioned in the center of the brain close to the hormone-producing *pituitary gland*, which is in contact with other areas of the brain that influence our consciousness and personality. The third eye chakra is also linked to the *pineal gland*, which influences our physiological rhythm and internal "clock" (circadian rhythm).

When the dynamic energy of the third eye chakra is activated and balanced, the rest of the brain functions optimally making this chakra particularly interesting in breathing exercises and meditation. The properties associated with the third eye chakra are transparency in the internal as well as the external vision, higher intuitive perception, wisdom, spirituality and creative intelligence. From an anatomical point of view it makes good sense that we should be able to access the pituitary gland by closing our eyes and "looking inward", because the two large nerve fibers of the eyes cross each other exactly in the area where the pituitary gland is located. By focusing awareness and energy on the third eye chakra you can manipulate the pituitary gland and its activity.

You have probably noticed Indians marking the "third eye" chakra with a colored dot. They often do this before they go to a temple or go on a long travel. The purpose is to make people they meet focus their attention and mental energy on the third eye chakra where it can be absorbed by the brain.

Collectively, the seven chakras symbolize different planes of consciousness. The higher they are located in the body, the higher the level of consciousness they represent. In other words at the bottom you find the primitive instincts, in the middle there is human behavior and towards the top are the more intellectual and divine aspects. To grow to a higher consciousness and develop as a human, you have to be able to arouse the force of your basic instinct to enable prana to rise freely upward towards the brain. If you wish to avoid it from running wild, it is important to regulate the intensity and direction of prana. For this purpose several body locks are used.

Small and large body locks

Various larger body locks (*bandhas*), which are muscle contractions in different areas of the body, are used in yoga. Likewise smaller body locks (*mudras*), are small changes in the limbs or organs such as the fingers, eyes or the tongue, are applied.

A shared feature of the locks is that they strengthen concentration and meditation by controlling the flow of prana.

There are three large body locks in particular that can be advantageous. They can be used separately, but when used at the same time, they are referred to as *Maha Bandha*, which means *Great Lock*. Apart from aiding in concentrating prana and stirring the sleeping energy in the body, *kundalini*, the *Great Lock* is also applied during breath holds, because it "locks" the air in your lungs.

The first bandha is the *Root Lock* that is performed by contracting the rectum to influence the inner and outer sphincter. In addition, the perineum area has to be lifted a bit. This is an important lock, because it stimulates the lower branch of the parasympathetic nervous system that extends from the spine in the lower part of the body. Stimulating the entire soothing nervous system in an optimal and balanced way.

The second bandha is the *Abdominal Lock*, and is performed by drawing the abdomen and navel towards the spinal column and then lifting it upwards. Because of a negative pressure within, the abdomen, diaphragm and all the internal organs are sucked up between the ribs. A person performing the *Abdominal Lock* will thus appear extremely thin. This bandha is spectacular and drives prana up along the spine. Only the exercise where the abdominal muscles rotate massages the internal organs to the same extent, improving digestion and strengthening the diaphragm. Even the heart is given a thorough massage.

The third bandha is the *Throat Lock*, which is performed by pressing the chin down towards the small depression just above the sternum making the chin and the two collar bones meet, locking the throat. The throat lock brings prana to a halt and directs it downwards to unite it with the upwards flowing prana in the chest area. Besides concentrating prana and activating dormant body energy, the *Throat Lock* is very effective during breath holds because air flow through the throat is inhibited and the lungs are cut off.

Apart from the bandhas – the large body locks – a set of mudra exists – small body locks. A mudra often used together with the *Great Lock* is the *Sambhavi Mudra*. In this lock focus and thought is directed towards the third eye chakra by looking cross-eyed upwards and inwards to pro-

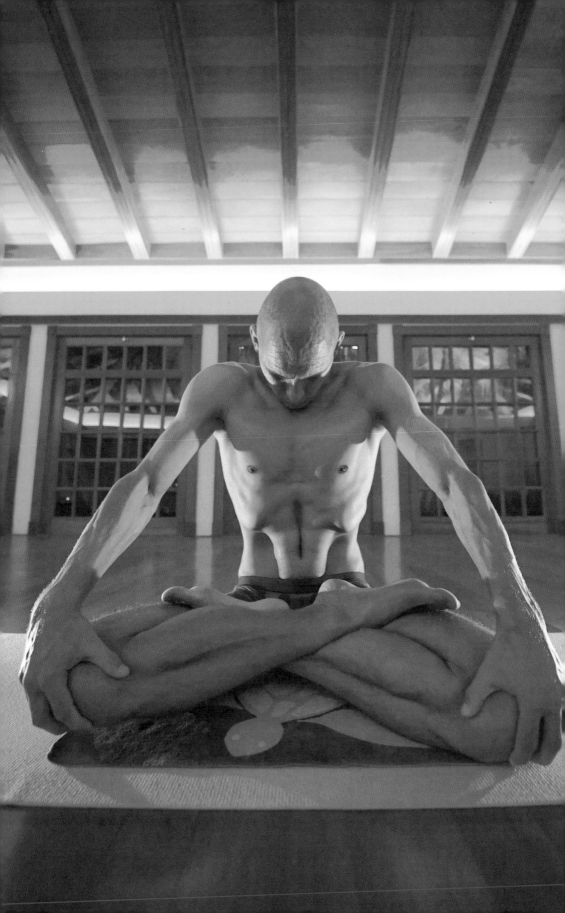

mote relaxation, concentration and meditation. Another small mudra is the well-known yoga position where the thumb and index finger join to form a ring with the palm of your hand pointing downwards, this is called the *Jnana Mudra*. It influences the psyche and symbolizes wisdom and intuitive knowledge. When the palm of your hand points upward, the lock is termed *Chin Mudra* and symbolizes an expanded consciousness. These two mudras are useful during meditation.

The final mudra I will mention is the *Kechari*, which in its ultimate form is one of the most difficult, effective and least known body lock of them all. Kechari exists in two varieties – a simple and an ultimate version. The "small" kechari is described as follows:

"Pursuing any livelihood, in any location, a yogi may practice nabho mudra.
Turn the tongue upwards, inhale and hold the breath.
This is nabho mudra; it destroys all diseases."

GHERANDA SAMHITA

The simple kechari is applied in connection with various asanas and pranayamas and is performed simply by turning the tongue backwards and pressing gently towards the soft palate. Its effect is beneficial to the heart, lungs and brain as a set of nerve fibers in the tongue as well as the palate is connected to these organs and thereby are soothed. In particular, the important vagus nerve is influenced. This is especially significant when you practice advanced pranayama exercises where the breath is held for a longer period of time.

To learn the ultimate kechari requires a good deal of practice, but the benefits you can gain are of many. During my stay in Rishikesh in Northern India in 2004, my teacher, Yogi Rakesh Ji, showed me this kechari several times where he forced his tongue into the nasal cavity. Every morning at sunrise I performed a set of exercises that massaged my tongue, made it stronger and stretched it. In brief, I performed "gymnastics" with my tongue. I pulled it to the side against the teeth in the lower jaw, gradually cutting the ligament below the tongue. I would clean the tongue with my fingers and a little cloth prior to the exercises, and as soon as it was dry, it was easy to grab with both hands and hold onto. Even a small amount of saliva on the tongue made it slippery as an eel and impossible to handle.

The Throat, Abdominal and Root Lock are performed at the same time in the Great Lock (Maha Bandha).

If yoga is of secondary importance to you, you obviously do not have to aim for the ultimate kechari. However, the importance of performing kechari with perfection is stressed repeatedly in the old scriptures. Kechari is particularly important because the tongue can be used to stimulate areas in the brain that control our hormone production, notably the pituitary gland. By controlling the area where the energy channels ida, pingala and sushumna meet (the third eye chakra), you gain control over the part of the nervous system that the will cannot control.

Accordingly, focusing your attention on the area between the eyebrows is very common in yoga because it creates balance and peace in the mind.

Another advantage of kechari is the ability to change the flow of air through your nostrils without using the fingers. The tip of the tongue can shut off the air flow through one nostril at a time. In this way you will be able to choose to breathe through either the left or right nostril. Finally, during breath holds it is possible to remove the urge to breathe and stop the natural contractions of the diaphragm with kechari – even though you have held your breath for a long time.

Cool or warm energy?

It may possibly seem a bit drastic that there is such a great focus on the many cleansing techniques, chakras and different body locks in yoga. Would it not suffice to just take deep breaths? The answer to this question lies in pranayama which is not only breath control, but also a method whereby the breath can be used to control the energy in the body. To understand the profound wisdom that yoga is based on, it is helpful to take a closer look at the symbolic explanations to the concepts previously addressed.

As described earlier, the energy channel of ida takes off from the left nostril. Ida is symbolized by the moon and thus represents a cool and calming energy. In effect, the body becomes passive, relaxed and receives rest. In contrast, the pingala in the right nostril is the warm energy from the sun that activates and stimulates our organism.

Do these two opposing energy systems not remind us of something we have encountered before? Yes, the two branches of the autonomous nervous system that modern science has named the parasympathetic and sympathetic pathways. Just as the case was with the different chakras corresponding to our hormone producing glands and nerve centers, the thousand-year-old Indian knowledge on the double-acting function of the nervous system bears witness to a fantastic intuitive understanding of the human body and mind. Not only in a theoretical sense, but also of its function, because it is made clear that you can influence your own existence by grasping the very fine axis of life that is breath.

Modern science is actually becoming aware of the fact that our nervous system and oxygen consumption differs when we breathe through the right or left nostril, and it will be interesting to follow what future studies may reveal.

According to this, ida (the moon) is the soothing parasympathetic pathway, while pingala (the sun) is the activating sympathetic pathway that keeps us alert and prepares us for "combat". When these two parts of the nervous system – sun and moon - are brought into balance by the breath, energy will be able to flow freely throughout the body. The brain will calm down, work harmoniously and effectively and will prepare for a higher level of consciousness.

This is the ultimate purpose of yoga and pranayama. And when there is a perfect balance between the two nostrils, samadhi (place of unity) can be experienced.

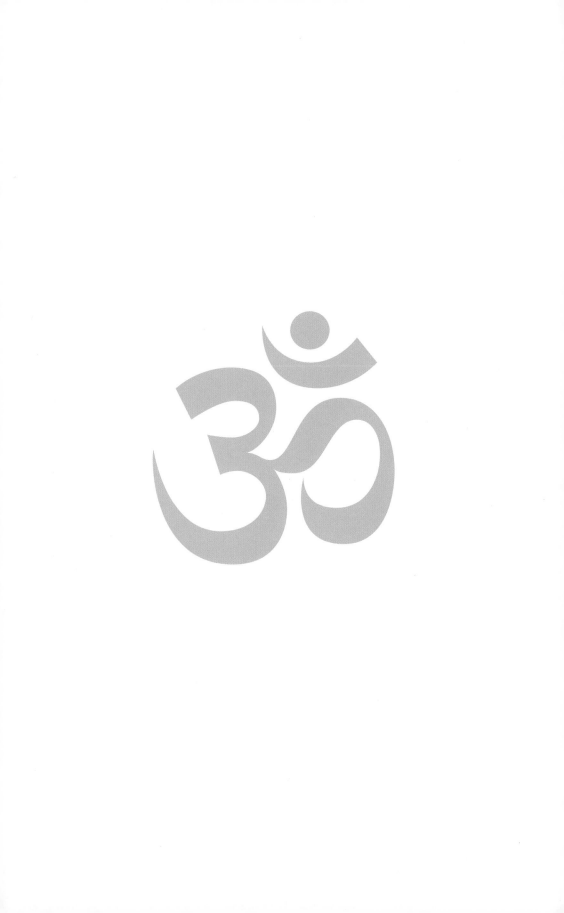

Exercises

Genuine yoga breath

The following exercises can be performed while lying on your back (*Relaxed Position*). You can also sit cross-legged on the floor, as long as you maintain a straight back.

Read through the exercises first and look at the illustrations. Practice the exercises alone or with a friend.

1) *YOGA BREATHING*

Seeing that you by now have reached a greater understanding of your natural breath, you will be able to work on modifying and optimizing it. This is done by learning the complete yoga breath, which is made up of three components: abdominal breathing, chest breathing and clavicular breathing. Place one hand on your abdomen and the other on your chest. Consciously inhale deep down into your "stomach" so that the hand on your abdomen moves upwards, and at the same time avoid moving the hand on your chest. Make sure that you are completely relaxed, especially in your shoulders, neck, tongue and forehead. If you feel like it, you can have a little smile on your lips – perhaps just an inner smile - like in the other exercises. If you find it difficult to separate the movement in your stomach from the chest, you can strap a belt tightly around your rib cage, and then you will not be able to use the muscles in your chest easily. Inhale, make your stomach swell, exhale and try to make the movements as slow and controlled as possible. After having filled the lower part of your lungs ("stomach") proceed by filling up the chest (the belt removed). This will lift the hand on your chest. The last part of the inhalation is performed in the upper part of the chest by lifting the collar bones a little. This completes the perfect yoga breath, which ends with a passive release of the air in your lungs starting from the top of your lungs and ending with the air in your "stomach", preparing you for another breath. It is important not to create tensions in the shoulders and neck by forcing air into the lungs, but to make the transition from the stomach to chest to collar bone as soft and smoothly as possible. The less energy you use, the more accurate the exercise has

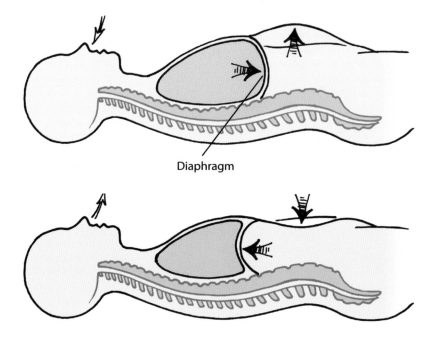

Diaphragm

The diaphragm is lowered and the stomach is pushed upwards (top figure).
The diaphragm returns to its initial position and the stomach flattens (below).

been performed. The purpose is to inhale as much air as possible with the least amount of effort. If you find it too difficult or strenuous to inhale the last bit of air by lifting the collar bone, then skip this last part of the breath, because it is more important that you use the diaphragm (may feel like the "stomach") and chest. The exercise can also be performed whilst sitting (e.g. at work, at meetings, in the bus), but because the muscles of the loin and stomach are keeping the spine upright, it is not quite as easy to lower the diaphragm and distend the stomach.

However, it is still a fantastic exercise, and it provides a thorough massage of the organs of the abdominal cavity – especially the liver and stomach that lie directly below the diaphragm. If you perform the exercise (gently) after your lunch break, you will enhance your digestion - which you will probably be able to feel and hear – try it! As mentioned, this breathing method is called yoga breathing, but it is nothing more than a natural and healthy breath. Practice this conscious breath as often as possible – you will be doing yourself a great favor. The most remarkable is that you will be changing your unconscious breath by practicing the yoga breathing, and this will strengthen your entire nervous system as well as influence your body, mind and soul.

2) *YOGA BREATHING WITH ABDOMINAL TENSION*

An often disregarded but important detail of training the breath is a pre-stressing of the lower part of the abdomen (below the navel). If you breathe exclusively down into the stomach, over time it can have consequences for the internal organs. Breathing solely with the top of your lungs is not desirable either, since it will result in less oxygen to the body and lead to stress and tension. The object is then to find an appropriate balance, and an abdominal tension is beneficial, because it serves to maintain the position of the internal organs while at the same time exposing them to a favorable pressure that increases their function. Place a hand on your belly just below the navel and try to breathe with your stomach only, but without making your hand move. It is not easy, but when you learn how to control the right muscles and coordinate them with the breathing, it will work by itself. Take your time and be patient. When yoga breathing is practiced in this way, it has a beneficial effect on your entire body.

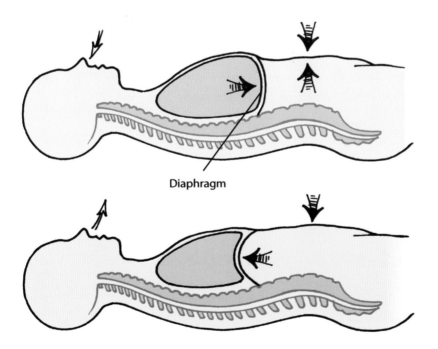

Diaphragm

The diaphragm is lowered but a slight tension in the abdominal muscles partly prevents the stomach from moving upwards (top figure). The diaphragm returns to its initial position and presses air out of the lungs aided by the muscular tension in the abdomen (below).

3) *TRAINING THE DIAPHRAGM*

The diaphragm is possibly the most important muscle you will ever be acquainted with. That is why it is useful to get to know it better and specifically train this muscle. Continue with yoga breathing, but try to force air out of the lungs by means of your muscles. Use the abdominal muscles, as if you are about to blow your nose, but do it slowly. Rest a hand on your belly and increase the frequency of your breaths to make the hand bob up and down. Do not use the chest during this exercise – only the diaphragm ("stomach"). Also try to fill as much air as you can into the lower part of your lungs and stretch your stomach to a greater extent by pushing the diaphragm down. Do not attempt to push too much, because it can cause discomfort or dizziness. Try to lift your "stomach" up between your ribs. You can do this by performing a little "swoop" or by "sucking" it up, while you are holding your breath. Lift and lower your diaphragm 10-20 times in a row. This is an excellent way to strengthen and supple the diaphragm, and at the same time it provides a gentle and healthy massage to your visceral organs, which will improve your digestion. Even your heart will be given a soft and comfortable massage from below in this exercise. Also try to perform the same "swoop" after exhaling. If it feels uncomfortable with empty lungs, just leave some air in the lungs.

In time you can combine ordinary *Yoga Breathing* and *Yoga Breathing with Abdominal Tension* with the following three locks:

> Sambhavi Mudra – maintain focus or your "inner eye" on the third eye chakra.
> Jnana or Chin Mudra – make a circle with the thumb and index finger and press them slightly together.
> "Little" Kechari Mudra – bend the tongue backwards and press it slightly towards the soft palate.

You can add them separately or do them all together.

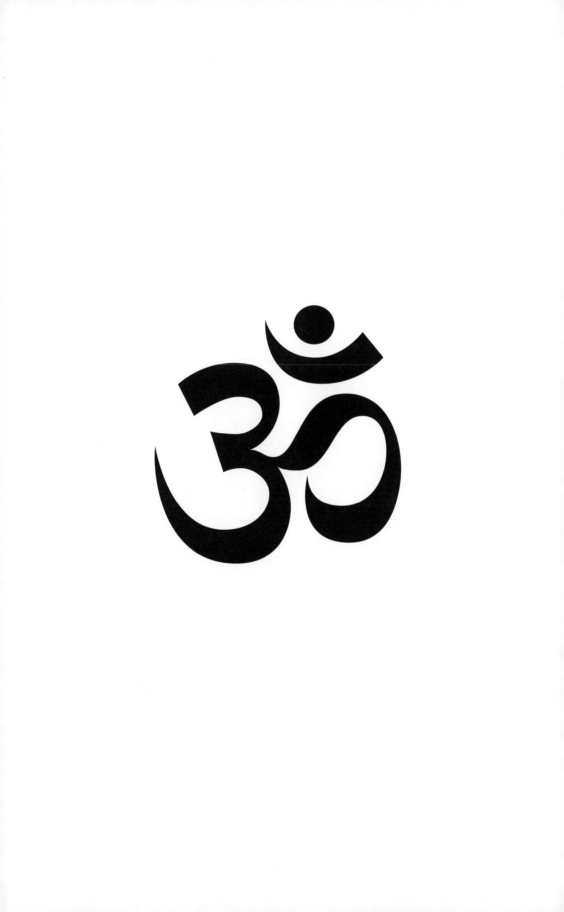

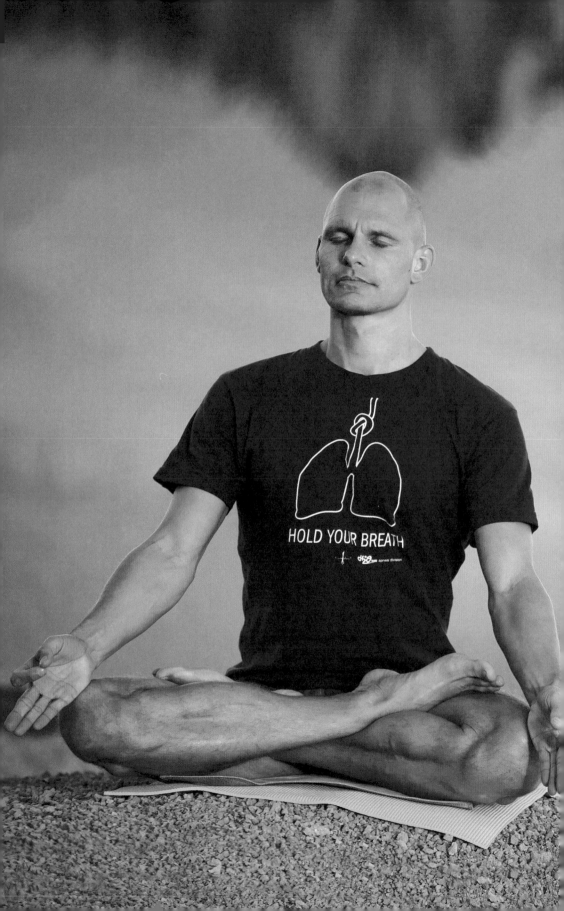

Sustained breathing

Holding your breath on land and in water

The natural pause

You may not be aware of how important holding your breath is. Without a natural pause between inhalation and exhalation, your breath would be abrupt and dissonant, so it is worthwhile to take a closer look at this pause. It is by no means necessary to be able to hold your breath for a long time to attain a soothing effect in the body and mind, but you should be able to feel comfortable with the exercise and relax completely. Now try to hold your breath – five seconds, ten seconds or perhaps even a minute. Close your eyes and direct your senses inwards. You might even be able to feel your heart or at least your pulse which you do not sense during the day. After a brief period of adapting, it is easy to improve your breath holding, and when you gain control over your breath holds you will learn more about yourself.

> "Just as lions, elephants and tigers are gradually controlled, so the prana is controlled through practice. Otherwise the practitioner is destroyed."
>
> HATHA YOGA PRADIPIKA

When you practice breathing through pranayama, the fourth element of yoga, it is vital to control life force energy (prana) and so controlling the breath is essential. The pause between inhalation and exhalation is termed *kumbhaka*, and it is a true art to extend this pause as much as possible. The highest form of pranayama is when the breath stops spontaneously. Even though the breath is literally "held", the aim is to make breathing stop and cease by itself, and so it is not intended to be a strenuous process. This state is termed *kevala kumbhaka*.

You may have experienced kevala yourself, but not been aware of it. Remember a very beautiful, overwhelming or surprising experience, and recall the spontaneous pause in your breathing where the moment is stretched unknowingly. In English we describe this phenomenon as becoming breathless. It simply means that for a moment you forget to breathe.

How do you hold your breath?

I have often been asked how I manage to hold my breath for so long – around nine minutes. In the light of yoga it is easier to comprehend, because it boils down to controlling the mind and gaining control over the autonomic nervous system that the will usually has no power to control. There is a world of difference between "holding your breath" and becoming one with the breath hold.

> "It is not because things are difficult that we do not dare;
> it is because we do not dare that they are difficult."
>
> SENECA

The art of holding the breath is to physically and mentally create a pause in which you simply do not breathe. To "hold your breath" suggests a strenuous task, whereas to "leave it be" is passive and effortless. When you do not either breathe or hold your breath, but rather just take a break, the mind can relax, and it is at the surface of this quiet lake of thoughts that the soul and intuition can reflect or shine through. Just as in yoga there are many different paths that lead to enlightenment in samadhi, so there are many different techniques and methods in freediving that can lead to a higher level of consciousness.

To be good at breath holding it is crucial to be able to forget or dissolve time. This state can be achieved through flow where you become one with your actions, or during a form of trance in meditation where you "forget yourself" – similar to when you are lost in your thoughts. The last thing to do whilst breath holding is to look at your watch or think about the time, because when you focus on time, it will also exist in your mind.

To consciously leave your consciousness, is one way of holding the breath, because if you yourself are not present this is easy to do. A neutral level of consciousness and control has to be maintained. When I perform long breath holds, I have an ability to be in a form of passive consciousness with a small "light channel" open to the external environment. The light channel is like a fine thread and constitutes my "safety line" exactly like your ears do when you sleep.

The correct physical tension and mental tranquility
are important elements in training and competition.

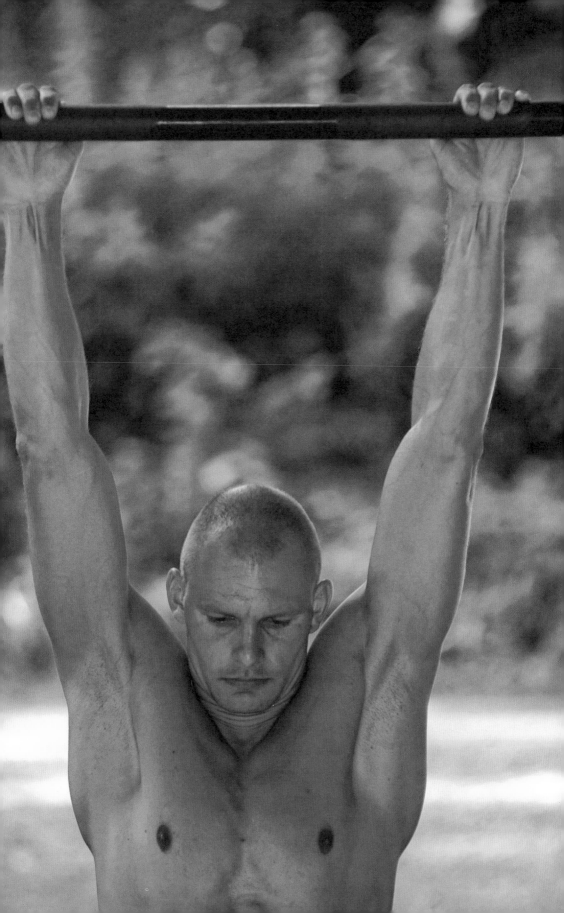

When you are in a deep sleep you do not hear anything, not even loud music, or should we say you hear everything but do not register it, because your senses are dormant. You react only to warnings - if your name is shouted out, or if the alarm clock rings. You have probably tried to wake up just before the alarm, so even though your consciousness has been "turned off", you have a kind of floating consciousness that lies above your normal level of consciousness. In the same way I have trained the ability to "return" on my own just before I terminate my dive.

Dissolve your thoughts

I would like to present a couple of examples on how I perform breath holds and what I experience. However, I will first answer another question I have often been given, namely, what my thoughts are during the long breath holds. This question is quite relevant, and I can understand why people wonder, but it is a very difficult question to answer unequivocally. The best answer must be that it is not important what you think, but how you think.

Various techniques are available to manage your stream of thoughts. You can actively try to eliminate negative thoughts that make you angry, sad or agitated by replacing them with positive or neutral thoughts. Similarly, you can try to suppress the negative thought by focusing on a positive state of mind. Reducing the speed of your thoughts also puts you in a more tranquil mode. Another approach is to passively imagine your thoughts as a series of trains that pass you on a platform. If you like you can board a carriage (a thought) and investigate it. What does it look like? If an unpleasant thought appears, just let it pass. Do not become agitated or try to throw the thought away. If it will not disappear, let it stay, and smile at it.

This exercise is a good mindfulness meditation where you consciously observe and accept the thoughts that appear without judging or analyzing them. Your thoughts can move on different levels, and you can teach yourself several different techniques of imagery and meditation. By improving your ability to observe and be attentive to your thoughts, you will in time be able to give your brain an effective massage, control your wandering thoughts, and create new positive ones.

There is much to learn about yourself by listening to your body "talking" to you. By increasing the awareness of your body and mind, you will connect to yourself in a new and different way, and thereby reach a higher level of relaxation, concentration and meditation. You have to simply be, or become one with yourself. Viewing meditation from this angle, you realize that it has nothing to do with being "religious" or as something wrapped in mystery and rituals, but is instead a way of thinking that is natural to all humans. And that it can be trained.

Sometimes I try to dissolve "normal" thought and focus on the movements of my body or its position instead. The heart is a central organ to be able to sense and control, and during my best dives I can feel my heart intensively. It beats in a very comfortable and soft way and its vibrations, or sounds if you like, completely absorb my mind. When you attain a good contact with your heart, learn to listen to it and are able to influence it significantly, you will quickly become good at holding your breath.

Another little amusing technique I sometimes use is the ability to rotate my body in my mind. When I lie face down and perform breath holding in water, I imagine my body slowly rotates 90 degrees around its longitudinal axis to make me lie upright. After having rotated slowly back to neutral position, I turn 90 degrees to the other side. Naturally, I do not move an inch, but it feels exactly as if I am lying on my side in the water.

A helpful piece of advice is to close your eyes. Besides saving oxygen on unimportant visual stimuli, it is easier to control your thoughts and thus the reactions of your body, when you turn your gaze inwards. When you travel to your inner universe, you will learn a lot of new and exciting things about yourself. In addition, you will detach yourself from the surroundings that are often distracting in your everyday life. If you are constantly stuck in the surrounding world, how are you ever going to relax and recharge your battery?

Breath holding in water

The famous quotation, "It is much better down there" from the movie *The Big Blue* in many ways sums up the essence of freediving where you hold your breath in water. As soon as you dive below the surface, you enter another universe and turn your gaze inwards. When you stop breathing and slowly fall down into the dark and quiet deep, you travel back to a state you know very well but do not remember - the time when you were weightless and comfortable in your mother's womb. The memories from the beginning of your life where you floated around in a little water-filled tank to the constant sound of a beating heart lie deep within your brain or spinal cord. A time in your life when the notion of

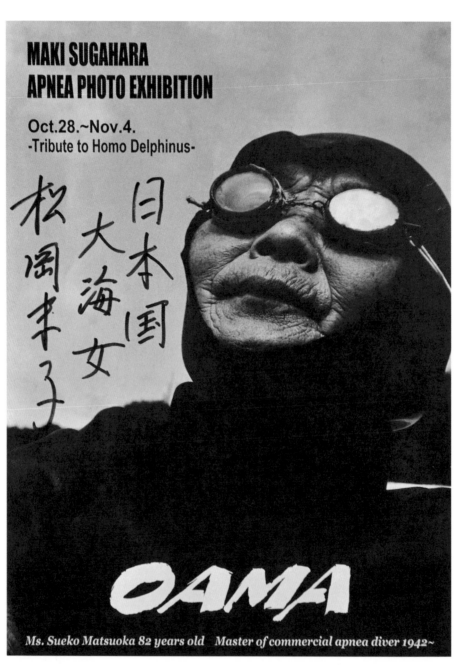

**MAKI SUGAHARA
APNEA PHOTO EXHIBITION**

Oct.28.~Nov.4.
-Tribute to Homo Delphinus-

日本国
大海女
松岡末子

OAMA

Ms. Sueko Matsuoka 82 years old   Master of commercial apnea diver 1942~

When I had the honor of meeting Ms. Sueko Matsuoka she was 82 year old. She has been working as a professional ama diver (pearl diver) in Japan since 1942 and had not had a sick day in more than 60 years. She still dives more than four hours a day and she intends to do so for many years to come. The story of her life is one of the most life-affirming and inspiring I have ever heard.

linear time line had not been introduced and where all your needs were fulfilled.

It is impossible to express the experiences you have below the surface with words, when water gently caresses your face and body, the pulse decreases and your brain relaxes. You are immediately cut off from the stress and hustle of everyday life when you are below the surface – there are no noisy telephones or SMS messages, no inboxes full of mail, no electrical bills, or other trivialities of everyday life taking up time and energy. There is nothing connecting you to the surface but the same withheld breath that connects you to life. There is only you and a growing pressure on your chest that feels like a loving hug and the vibrations from the deep quiet tone of the sea. It is quite possible that this deep quiet tone is none other than the mantra Om, the sound of the universe, trickling life into every cell of your body.

In professional freediving you compete over who can hold the breath the longest – you "stress" the body and mind to a degree that people might consider extreme. Thus self-insight and the ability to relax are extremely important. Luckily, you can employ these qualities with equal success when you have returned to the surface of the earth. This is why applying freediving techniques to many situations in a hectic everyday life is so pleasing and beneficial.

If you are engaged in water activities such as surfing, kayaking, rafting etc., a basic knowledge of how breath holding affects you is highly relevant. This especially applies to people who spent time below the surface engaged in SCUBA diving, training of aquatic animals, lifeguarding and the like, since circumstances might change instantaneously. Knowing how to hold ones breath is a big safety factor, which can help you avoid panic and stay calm even during dangerous events.

"He who knows pranayama and kevali is the real Yogi. What can he not accomplish in this world, who has acquired success in kevali kumbhaka?"

GHERANDA SAMHITA

Indeed breath holding is a true art that can do you a wealth of good. In many ways it is rather complicated, but it is also quite simple and only requires that you do not give it too much thought. You can reasonably compare breath holding to a simple physical balancing act. If you are walking on a bar or a beam and your balance is working, it is easy. It is when you start thinking about what you are doing or doubt that you can hold your balance that you fall. Freediving is exactly the same. So listen to your body!

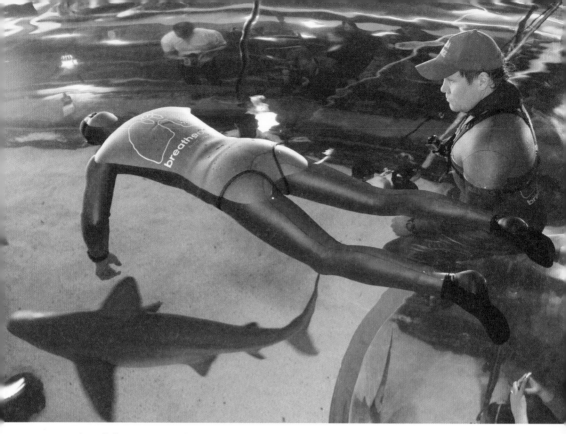

The ability to control your body and mind and enter a state of flow can lead to peak performance in stressful situations.

On April 1. 2010, I reached the epitome of breath holding, when I became the first person to pass the magical 20-minute barrier. The dive was done in a tank with tropical sharks after inhaling pure oxygen and was an official Guinness World Record. Total dive time was 20 minutes and 10 seconds and during all this time I used different techniques of concentration and meditation such as body relaxation, childhood memories and the ability to forget myself. In my mind, the dive was of a more mental than physical nature and the ability to suppress my breathing reflex for such a long time was deeply rooted in my belief that it was actually possible.

The noble art of breath holding

Freediving is also called *apnea*, a Greek word meaning "without air". You probably know the concept of sleep apnea which is an illness where the body simply "forgets" to breathe during sleep.

Over the course of history freediving has been used for various purposes. In Denmark enormous piles of clamshells have been found during excavations of Stone Age settlements, a witness to the fact that our ancestors collected food below the surface. Along the Mediterranean Sea, freediving is still employed to collect sponges, and in Japan the famous breath holders, the Ama divers, dive and collect pearls, seaweed and shellfish from the deep using only one breath or air. During a tour around the world in 1996, I visited the Badjao, the Sea Gypsies that are boat dwellers in the Celebes and Sulu Sea between Borneo and the Philippines. Badjao are nomads of the sea and seldom go ashore. They live in houseboats and in stilt-houses in the sea. When I came to Cebu port, the young badjao no longer dived for sponges or fish but dived for shiny coins thrown in the water by tourists.

Today freediving is practiced widely as a leisure sport such as in snorkeling or spearfishing. Anybody can enter the sea and experience the colorful animals and enjoy the peaceful feeling of weightless freedom that the water bestows.

Freediving has become more and more widespread on a professional level over the last 50 years with different kinds of competitions. In the last 10 years it has experienced a true renaissance. This is partly due to a greater organization of the professional freediving community, leading to greater attention by the media.

Perhaps the most important reason is that freediving matches current trends where more and more people wish to know themselves better and come closer to nature - thus becoming part of the holistic lifestyle that freediving shares with yoga.

"It all began when my father needed Stig's autograph for my birthday. So he sent a letter where he wrote about how fond of water and diving I was. I received a letter from Stig where he offered me a personal course at Aarhus Freediving Club. I was thrilled and enrolled as a member in the club after the course and have been there ever since. I could not swim even 50 meters dynamic before I started freediving, but I do more than 100 meters today. I have also bought a fancy underwater camera to take pictures of all the fascinating animals I meet below the surface."

Marcus Møller Bitsch, 16 year old freediver

**In freediving one golden rule applies:
NEVER dive alone!**

My 8´40 record

I will now invite you to join me below the surface in a dive I performed, and go through the different stages of the dive. I hope you will recognize aspects of the body's reaction and the holistic line of thought from yoga philosophy that you have already been acquainted with.

> "The feeling of slipping without falling"
>
> THE BIG BLUE

The dive took place at the international competition, Aarhus Triple Challenge in the summer of 2007 and lasted 8 minutes and 40 seconds. It was registered as the best dive on the World Ranking List that year, and I was awarded the prize "World Freediving Award 2007". The dive was a so-called *Static Apnea* breath hold where I lay motionless in water holding my breath just below the surface.

Preparatory breathing

Before a competitive dive I spend about four minutes sitting with my eyes closed and breathe quietly. I kneel in shallow water (the diamond posture), keep my back straight in a natural position, making sure that the chest is open, and listen to my deep, harmonious and slow breath. I am mentally focused on being relaxed, having an inner smile and feeling light. Three minutes before the dive, I breathe a bit deeper, always through the nose. Two minutes before, I begin to breathe more heavily and exhale through the mouth, which I shape as a funnel. This is called "purge breathing" because the mouth acts as a valve and creates a higher pressure in the lungs, which makes the alveoli open up like flowers to allow blood to absorb more oxygen.

My eyes are still closed, and if I open them, I do not notice anything, but just watch passively – like when you are lost in your own thoughts. The last 30 seconds before the dive I breathe even more heavily and have a single big yawn. I have trained the ability to yawn on command, and as you know a yawn has a lovely, pleasant and soothing effect. Furthermore, it is a signal to the body and mind that it is time to become fully relaxed.

> *When you hold your breath and are in deep*
> *meditation, you can forget both time and yourself.*

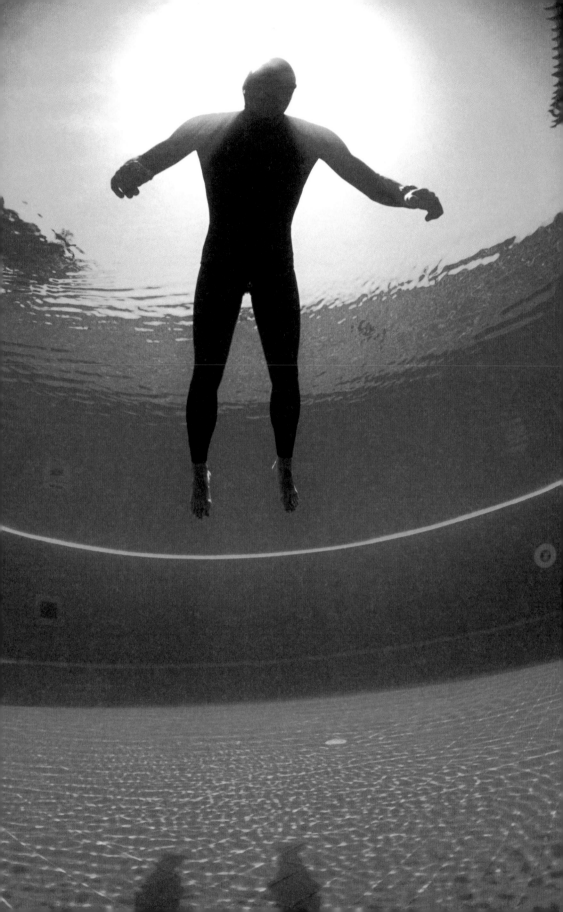

I use the full *Yoga Breathing* where the "stomach" (the diaphragm) and the chest are utilized optimally. The last exhalation is deeper and longer than usual. I put a little smile on my lips and slowly, with control, fill up the lungs starting from the bottom. When I cannot fill more air into my lungs, I carry out a final motion that I developed many years ago, and to my surprise have not seen other freedivers perform. When I press lightly against my thighs with my fingers, the pressure in my lungs drop for a moment, because the position of the diaphragm changes, and by relieving the rib cage I can inhale even more air into the top of my lungs and throat by means of the collar bones.

Afterwards I "pack" a few additional liters of air into the lungs by using the tongue as a piston. This is a well-known freediving technique, but it is not utilized anywhere else, which is a shame, because "packing" can be useful in many other situations. We will address that topic later in *Therapeutic Breathing*. I pack 12 times and put the diving mask on at the same time, before slipping into the water to the countdown of the judge.

Pulse drop and moonlight

The pressure in the packed lungs is high, but it feels right, and only a few seconds pass before I feel the diving reflex initiate, and my pulse drops. I make sure that my neck and particularly my tongue are completely relaxed and create a weak pressure between the throat and the underside of the tongue to make it press slightly against the back of the mouth. This creates an airtight "lock" that together with a weak *Throat Lock* keeps the air in the lungs.

After a brief period of time a clear disc of light appears before my inner sight. As previously described, different techniques such as relaxation, imagery, concentration and mediation can be employed. You can have various thoughts or recall memories from your childhood or holidays with your family, partner and friends. Or you can try to recreate beautiful moments or emotions you have had below the surface with oscillating ocean currents, dancing seaweeds and corals, or perhaps recall beautiful animals you have met below the surface – dolphins, sharks, sea turtles or tiny colorful fish.

But during this dive there it is a little disc that takes up my mind. The light in the disc is cool and colored like the moon, and around it small rays of light blaze in the shape of lotus leaves. The colors change between blue and green with orange in the middle, very much like a little flame from a gas light. Now and then the surrounding light becomes brighter and glaring, as when you are underwater gazing up into the sun and light rays break through the surface in a dusty fan.

In retrospect I recall having experienced a similar color and disc twice in my life. Once, I experienced it during a night dive in the mid-90´s with my good friend and dive buddy Christoffer while lying on the bottom of Aarhus Bay gazing up into a starry sky that was lit by a large full moon. To those of you who have not experienced the moon from below the surface, I can tell you that it assumes a special and almost electrical gleam that you do not experience on land. The other occasion was during the Depth Freediving World Championship in Egypt in the Autumn of 2007 when I pulled myself down along a rope together with two Swedish freedivers to a depth of 80 feet wearing only a diving mask.

During the initial static performance, I entered the light disc and disappeared into my mind, completely absent from the pool and the dive. In connection with this, it is particularly interesting to mention the different phenomena that appear in the mind, when siddhis, the beneficial advantages of yoga, begin to take shape. When you have held your breath for a long time during yoga, you can see fog, smoke, hot winds, fire, fireflies, lightening, crystals or the moon.

Signals from the body

After roughly five minutes the first weak signs that the body wishes to breathe appear, but I defer the contractions of the diaphragm. After six minutes the stomach begins to move, but I try to make the contractions in the diaphragm as small and soft as possible. The contractions increase somewhat after seven minutes but are not unpleasant. I make sure my neck is relaxed and use my tongue to soften the contractions and the pressure in the lungs. After eight minutes the contractions begin to increase in strength, but I move them to the side of the body and go deeper and deeper into the contractions to relax.

Mentally, I am completely focused, almost in a trance. About eight minutes and 30 seconds into the dive my little internal alarm goes off denoting that it is time to emerge. After exactly 8 minutes and 40 seconds I gently surface while exhaling, take a deep breath and feel happy and well.

My first inhalation after a long breath hold is what is referred to as a "hook-breath", which consists of the air being held in the lungs while at the same time increasing pressure by tightening the diaphragm and abdominal muscles while keeping the throat and epiglottis closed. This technique is utilized by most elite freedivers because it elevates oxygen tension in the lungs and allows for the release of more oxygen into the blood. "Hook-breathing" was originally invented by fighter pilots during the Second World War in order to oxygenate the brain when experiencing a tremendous gravitational pull. Hereafter, the technique was almost forgotten and I believe it is only used actively by freedivers today. This is a shame because "hook-breathing" can be beneficial in many circumstances.

After the dive I smile and make sure to complete the proper protocol according to the rules, and wait to see whether the judges approve with a white card that officially recognizes the dive.

The path to your inner paradise

A freediver invents and constantly tests new methods, because it is the nature of the freediver to investigate and optimize in every possible (and impossible) way. The obvious reason is that only a limited amount of oxygen is available in a single breath. In general, top freedivers understand human and animal physiology and the mental processes well. Add respect for nature and the ability to combine and convert knowledge, experience, and intuition in order to produce results that, in the world of freediving, are measured in time, depth and length.

Freediving is a lifestyle rather than a sport. This explains why there is a focus on the spiritual aspects. Even if competitive freediving may seem driven by results, the relationship between the physical and the spiritual makes up the actual core of the sport. Key concepts are balance and harmony between the mind and the exterior world, between man and the universe.

I can confirm that a combination of long breath holds, complete relaxation and concentration/meditation generates a sensation of euphoria and rapture, which creates mental clarity that may rest in the body for hours or even days after a successful dive.

> "God is at the bottom of the sea and I dive to find him."
> ENZO MAIORCA

The freediving legend, Jacques Mayol, told the following story after a stay in India. He met a retired college professor who had given up his professional career and moved to a small cottage to practice yoga with the purpose of dissolving his ego. He was in his early sixties and with intensive training he managed to hold his breath for more than six minutes during his yoga exercises. After a brief introduction to the Valsalva maneuver, where you equalize the pressure in the middle ear, Jacques Mayol enticed him to swim to the bottom of a lake. In his first attempt the professor stayed at the bottom of the lake for more than 6 minutes, and when he returned to the surface, he exclaimed, "You were right, Mr. Mayol... This is indeed a shortcut to Samadhi!" (Paradise).

> "Dear Stig,
> Being 76 years old, I have to nurse myself a lot. It is often a question about having the right philosophical attitude to maintain a positive mind under these circumstances. Breathing properly really becomes a genuine sport and the last and final activity of old people. All of us should practice our breathing to survive as comfortably as possible. In a way, to everybody life is a competition with yourself to endure difficulties and problems that worsen with every day and every year that passes. The more tired the "machine" is, the more often the "carburetor" has to be adjusted.
> Let me make a comparison. If you wish to adjust the carburetor in your car, you have to almost "strangle" the engine first, and thereupon turn gently in the opposite direction. You may say that we should do the same to our human "breathing-engine". Anytime in life, breath holding is the proper method to accomplish this. Of course, you have to learn to perform deep breaths and breathe properly (with your diaphragm) first to attain the desired level of relaxation. Only then may you visit your "second" breath by performing a prolonged breath hold. The small bobs and contractions in the diaphragm then become controlled reactions, and your anxiety and despair simply vanishes, when you start breathing again."

> Guy Ackermann, journalist and breathing enthusiast
> Hermance, Switzerland

A message from yoga

Freediving can be viewed as a mediator of our time between yoga and the modern knowledge-based society. The credit for bringing Eastern traditions into the Western world of freediving should be given to the aforementioned legendary French freediver, Jacques Mayol. If your freediving knowledge is sparse but the name "Jacques Mayol" still rings a bell, this may be due to the fact that you have seen Luc Besson's classical movie The Big Blue from 1988. The movie depicts a friendship between Jacques Mayol and his Italian rival Enzo Maiorca, and it drew significant attention to the world of freediving. At the same time the movie showed how attractive freedivers are to scientists, because these athletes can produce astonishing performances in controlled experiments.

The physiological changes that take place when you dive, such as the lowering of the heart beat and a change in the blood flow, can be described scientifically, whereas the feelings that flow through the body when you hold your breath in water have to be experienced to be understood. As in yoga, these experiences of a more mental and spiritual nature cannot be rationalized. You cannot understand them by reading about them – you have to jump in the water yourself!

> "I became aware of the power of breathing properly for the first time when I went freediving with Stig in the Red Sea. After performing breathing exercises for a couple of days I could hold my breath for more than 4 minutes in the water. The sensation of surplus mental energy and inner tranquillity was intoxicating."
>
> Bjarne Brynk Jensen, 43
> Company coach and consultant for the Winter Olympics in Vancouver 2010

Many parallels can be drawn between freediving and yoga. The shared objective is to optimize and improve all the physiological and mental processes by gaining self-understanding, self-control and self-discipline. In time this will create a deeper understanding and respect for human nature and the way humans interact with each other as well as with their environment. Particularly our breathing, which we share with all other beings, is important because we can accomplish the most incredible things when we pay attention to our breathing.

Many of the postures and breathing exercises in yoga are integrated from the animal kingdom, and this is also true of freediving. Not only the way we swim and the use of equalization techniques, but to a great extent how we hold our breath for a prolonged period of time. It is quite impressive what you can learn from simply observing and trying things out.

"I specifically recall a dive in a 50 meter pool. When I emerged because of low oxygen, Stig asked why I emerged so soon. It was merely my brain that wanted to breathe, but my body was capable of swimming much further. After some training I added more meters to the distance. I also began to swim a series of dives, and I actually liked it when I had recovered from the initial fright!"

Mette Jacobsen, 37
Five times Olympic competitor, 36 medals at EC and WC

Personal development

As in yoga, freedivers often demonstrate "supernatural" abilities - holding the breath for more than 10 minutes, diving below 200 meters etc. Naturally, there is nothing supernatural about it, and since, as opposed to yoga, there exists a competitive component in professional freediving, where the results are measured in meters and seconds, even the greatest sceptic has to recognize the results.

In this way freediving elegantly validates many of the myths of the old yoga scriptures. So it is not all mumbo jumbo and there is probably some truth to what was written regarding the notion that the ultimate control of the breath leads to ultimate control of the mind. My personal experience confirms this - let me add an example on how I have tried to bridge the gap between the physical and mental world.

In 2003 my dear friend and training partner, Peter Pedersen, broke a world record performing a 200-meter dive with fins. At the time it was quite unthinkable to dive beyond this point. The greater was the joy and surprise when I was the first to pass the magical 200-meter barrier at a large international competition in the Netherlands later that year. A few months earlier I had set up my first world record attempts to dive as deep and as far on one breath as humanly possible, without fins. I began to work with mental processes on setting up objectives, imagery and tension regulation.

Each morning I performed yoga, and the program often consisted of asanas (postures and stretching exercises), focusing on the breath, pranayama (breath control), relaxation, concentration, meditation and prayer. I was particularly absorbed in pranayama, and my control had progressed to the point where I could hold my breath for more than eight minutes. I was also in a pretty good physical condition with a cardiovascular fitness rating of VO2 Max above 60. I aimed at broadening my consciousness (and subconsciousness) by means of the concept which I call "mental plasticity".

I focused on transforming my mind and making it more adaptable to let my subconscious accept the images and thoughts I formed during my yoga sessions. I wanted my dreams and visions to become just as integrated as the rest of my body. The breath and long breath holds turned out to be excellent tools for strengthening and maintaining these images.

Concurrently, I spent a lot of time on getting to know my responses in stressful situations during maximum (long) training dives. Slowly but surely, I moved deeper and deeper down through different mental layers and got to know the subtle signals of the body. Each dive was like a world record attempt to me – it was never just for the fun of it, because I was very curious to investigate how far I could push my mental boarders by constantly going to the edge.

It became a game to act out my full potential, and it was merely a question of time before I had achieved the ability to control my entire nervous system to the point that pain no longer played a significant role. No matter how acidic my legs became, how my sight changed (tunnel vision, purple haze, black-white etc.), whether I had buzzing or ringing in my ears, and no matter how much my diaphragm pumped up and down, I maintained concentration and the joy of being in the water - which I love – and did my best.

In the end the pain was like a friend – the more pain, the more inner tranquillity I could reach. It was interesting to enter the pain and closely investigate the experience instead of feeling sorry for myself! I discovered and gradually developed an inner rhythm that I could focus on enabling me to disregard my body's reactions and surroundings.

Naturally, not all days were alike, and it was frustrating to break off a dive because concentration failed. But I also came to appreciate the dives that were interrupted and learned something positive from them. As a matter of fact, I probably learnt more from these dives, because they made me reflect on what had gone wrong - and why.

The good dives were obviously fantastic. The sensation of being able to dissolve or leave my body, timelessness, the warm flow, the inner sparkling energy, the extreme comfort and sensation of joy. These dives gave me a feeling of being on a mission and provided my existence with a profound meaning, while at the same time gave me the ability to focus 100% in a matter of seconds. You could say that relaxation, concentration and meditation fused to a higher level in these dives – a progression of results during each dive over time, and a regression to my deeper instincts and the values of my soul.

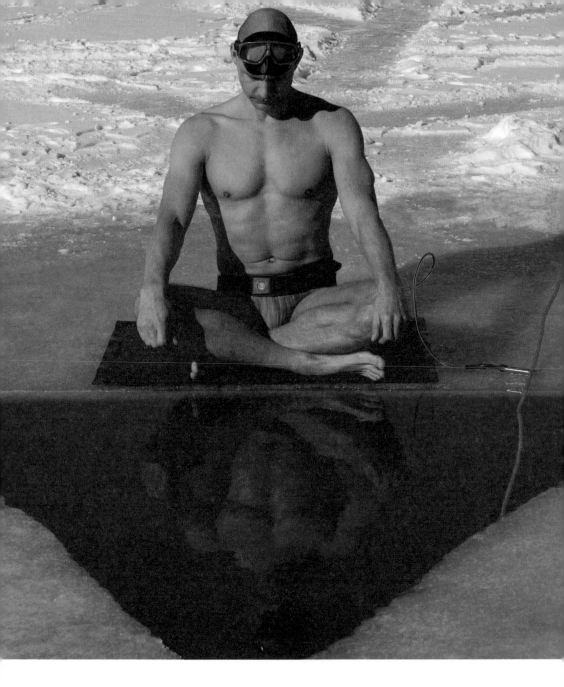

The ability to endure pain and focus completely on the task at hand came into full effect during my Guinness World Record under ice in March 2010. Equipped with only swimming trunks and goggles I held my breath and swam 236 feet (72 meters) under ice in a frozen lake. Even though the icy water was extremely cold and nearly paralyzed my body, I maintained a state of full attention and relaxation and ended the dive with a smile.

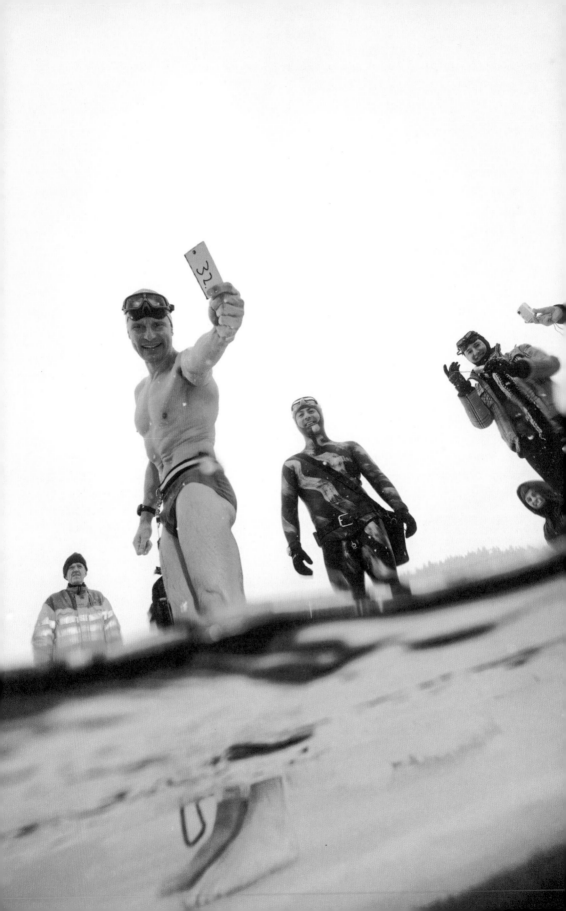

As in yoga, the last phase in freediving is spiritual – you wish to merge with your surroundings, usually the sea. The goal is not, as some may believe, to transform into a fish or a dolphin – you only wish to become a complete human being.

Extreme reactions

If you merely snorkel on the surface or dive a little when you go for a swim, there is no need to worry about the reactions of your body. You cannot suffer decompression sickness, which is a super saturation of nitrogen in your body caused by a higher nitrogen tension in your lungs. It is safe to swim around and watch fish, but remember never to swim or dive alone.

Some precaution, however, should be taken when you challenge your freediving skills, because when the body is pushed to the extreme a lot of physiological changes occur. If you perform multiple dives, it is a good rule of thumb to breathe at the surface three times longer than you spend below the surface. In this way you can avoid freediving decompression sickness. If you perform numerous dives in a row, you can become ill from freediving decompression sickness.

Even though this had been proven by the Danish physiologist Poul Erik Paulev in the sixties, many are not aware of the risk that exists when multiple or very deep dives are practiced. If you suffer decompression sickness as a freediver, the consequences are the same as for scuba divers. The gas tension of nitrogen rises, leading to the formation of tiny bubbles that can block blood vessels (e.g. in the brain) and thereby inhibit blood flow. Today the world's greatest freedivers have reached depths where oxygen (O_2), carbon dioxide (CO_2) and nitrogen (N_2) can become poisonous to the nervous system and can lead to trembles, paralysis or mental changes. Collectively, these phenomena are termed *narcosis*.

If you ignore the signals of your body, which I call "the little bell", you can experience a *samba* in freediving. A samba occurs when you have held your breath for too long and pushed your body beyond its limits leading to convulsions and an unclear mind due to the nervous system

The body reacts effectively on extreme conditions. During this deep dive through a hole in the ice at the Oslo Ice Challenge 2009, the diving reflex was particularly strong and the urge to breathe was completely absent.

being under pressure and low oxygen tension. It has been given the name "samba" because in some instances the convulsions may remind you of a samba dancer that shakes and moves.

When you completely ignore the warning signs of your body or are unable to react – e.g. if you are taken by a current during a deep dive – it is somewhat like passing an intersection when the traffic signals are red - and you can end up getting a *blackout* - meaning loss of consciousness. Neither a samba nor a blackout are desirable, but let me point out to you that there is no scientific evidence showing that they cause damage to the brain or any other part of the body – neither short- nor long-term, but more on this later.

It is worth noticing that even if you reach the point of unconsciousness, it does not mean that the brain or the body lacks oxygen. Many people are not aware of this vital point, or they forget how the body works. As long as the heart beats, oxygenated blood is directed into the system, even when the heart beats slowly, as it does during breath holds.

The loss of consciousness is a defence mechanism of the body showing that it is under an enormous pressure. Shutting down consciousness saves oxygen and energy and happens before actual damage to the brain occurs. Examples exist of people who have drowned for up to 30–40 minutes and have been revived with more or less no damage. Particularly, if the water is freezing cold, since it intensifies the diving reflex.

Your inner dolphin

Humans and other mammals have a *diving response* consisting of a set of reflexes that are activated when our face is cooled (such as by the water during a dive) or if we hold our breath. The diving reflex is a clever physiological mechanism enabling the body to tolerate a low level of oxygen. This is partly achieved by a lower heart beat and partly by a constriction of the peripheral blood vessels in the arms and legs to shunt blood to the vital internal organs like the heart and brain that require oxygen the most.

The changes in the body occur relatively quickly, within 30 seconds. The reflex is preventive because it is initiated before the level of oxygen becomes critically low. In addition the large amount of blood that accumulates in the blood vessels of the lungs acts as a protective measure, because fluids - as opposed to tissue and bones - cannot be compressed. The blood thus prevents the lungs from collapsing under the high pressure of the deep.

Another action of the diving response can be observed in infants when they are under water. The windpipe by the vocal chords spontaneously closes to prevent water from entering the lungs. This reflex is initiated as soon as there is contact with water. However, it disappears when the child reaches the age of roughly six months.

Recent investigations have shown that the spleen, which contains red blood cells, also plays a significant role during dives and breath holds. Following a number of dives, the spleen contracts and releases a large quantity of red blood cells to the circulatory system. Spleen contraction occurs much slower than the other diving reflexes. The release of more red blood cells allows more oxygen to be stored in the blood. Finally, the additional amount of blood cells allows the body to regain its normal balance faster after a prolonged breath hold. Popularly speaking, the spleen acts as a kind of "turbo" - during and after a long dive.

Diving mammals such as whales and seals naturally have a well-developed diving reflex to allow them to forage below the surface for extended periods of time. There are several reasons why the sperm whale, seals and elephant seals are excellent breath holders and can dive for more than an hour. Firstly, these animals have quite a lot of blood and a high concentration of blood cells which bind oxygen in the so-called *hemoglobin* protein. In addition, they have a higher concentration of an oxygen-binding molecule called *myoglobin* in their muscles. Have you ever seen whale or seal meat, and wondered why it is so dark? Myoglobin is the answer. A high content of iron in myoglobin colors the meat brown.

The diving mammals are also able to cool their brain down, which helps them during prolonged dives. Several studies show that seals can lower their body and brain temperature with up to 3 degrees Celsius, and thereby lower their metabolism and oxygen consumption dramatically. As opposed to humans, seals may completely shut off blood supply to the limbs and thus direct oxygenated blood to the lungs, heart and brain.

The Aquatic Ape Theory

It is quite striking how man resembles marine mammals by the possession of the same reflexes and physiological adaptations to life in water. This is not necessarily a coincidence, and a natural explanation could exist.

Water is very appealing to many people, and most children love water. As a matter of fact infants can swim and float, because of their thick layer of fat, natural kicking motion, and their inborn diving reflex, which prevents water from entering their lungs. It is reasonable to consider why a terrestrial being such as man is a relatively good swimmer, especially when we are compared to our closest relatives, the great apes.

The most prevalent theory of the evolution of modern man is that our ancestors became bipedal about five million years ago on the great open savannahs of Africa. In effect, our hands were liberated to handle weapons and other tools, but there are points that argue against the *Savannah Theory*.

To oppose this prevalent theory of our evolution, an alternative theory has emerged. Neither anatomically nor physiologically does man resemble a typical terrestrial animal. For instance, we have naked skin with a thick layer of subcutaneous fat instead of fur. Fur (or feathers) provides the best insulation in air, whereas fat is more effective in water. A long body and spine, a big head and a gait that does not seem natural suggests an entirely different animal group, namely the marine mammals.

Of course humans do not descend from dolphins or seals, but many common traits have lead to the *Aquatic Ape Theory*. According to this theory, which has been advocated by the zoologist Sir Alister Hardy and in particular the author Elaine Morgan, modern man evolved along the shores of Eastern Africa. This shoreline environment let to the development of traits advantageous in and near water. These early humans evolved bipedal gait, because they foraged in shallow water for clams and other food items, and developed their diving response diving for fish and other marine foods. This new food source was rich on omega-3 fatty acids, a major component of fish oil, leading to the development of a larger brain within a relatively brief period of time. Today, science shows that polyunsaturated fatty acids are important for the development of a healthy brain and a functional nervous system.

The ability to control the breath would have been essential during dives and combined with the complex brain the creation of an advanced language could have come about. A similar complex language exists in dolphins and whales, which are considered to be very intelligent animals. Indeed, the language is so complex that man has no idea what these animals are talking about. I have had the pleasure of accompanying a large group of Norwegian killer whales during a herring hunt just north of the Polar Circle, and from a short range I can bear witness to an extremely varied repertoire of sounds including clicks, whistles and sounds from a deep tone to a high pitch.

We cannot be certain of exactly how man evolved about five million years ago, but it is a fascinating and interesting thought that it could have been the ability to control the breath that fathered our advanced linguistic communication and thereby the social evolution of man.

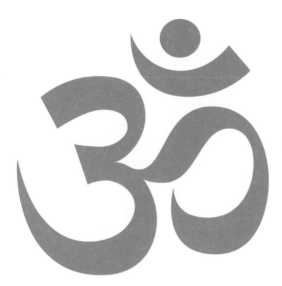

Exercises

You have now learnt to control your body and mind by means of relaxation and concentration exercises. You have also become more conscious of your breathing, and thereby gained better control over your breath. With these skills you are ready to explore the science of the breath, pranayama.

Pranayama in practice

Let us now engage profoundly in pranayama and the specific breathing techniques you are about to learn to enable you to get started with the exercises that will make you a true master of the noble art of breathing and breath holding.

As previously described, classic pranayama consists of three parts: inhalation, exhalation and the interposed pause (kumbhaka). When you hold your breath with your lungs full of air, it is denoted *antara kumbhaka*, and when the breath is held on empty lungs it is called *bahya kumbhaka*. The art of pranayama is to control the three phases of the breath, especially exhalation and breath holding.

When you commence pranayama, do not hold your breath, but let your inhalation and exhalation be of equal length (ratio 1:1). When you control your breath to the point where it flows harmonically, you can expand the exhalation to twice the time of the inhalation (ratio 1:2). It might take you a week to learn this, perhaps even a month! Subsequently, you can start to hold your breath between the inhalation and exhalation (ratio 1:1:1). When you have accomplished this, the ratio can be varied in a number of ways, but a very commonly applied ratio is 1:4:2: e.g. inhale 10 seconds, hold your breath 40 seconds and exhale 20 seconds. In this example one cycle will last 1 minute and 10 seconds.

Each exercise has many variations, but I will only examine the most simple and important here. It is a fundamental rule not to perform breath holds in the beginning. Thus there is no pause between the inhalation and the exhalation except for the natural pause that occurs when the breath changes direction. Furthermore, it is essential that this change in direction is performed as smoothly as possible. Imagine a soft curve that moves up and down in a wavy fashion. When you approach the "top" of your inhalation, take your time and make a slight pause. Then proceed with the exhalation in the same calm manner. Breathe similarly when you reach the "bottom" of your exhalation.

This may seem banal, but it is my experience that this curve is the most important thing to understand (and control) in order to create a perfect and harmonious flowing breath. If your breathing curve resembles peaky mountains, you are definitely doing something wrong. Try drawing your breathing curve yourself or ask a friend to draw the curve for you, preferably when you are not aware of it, because your breath will change as soon as you start thinking about it.

Pranayama includes a series of breathing exercises that have different effects on the body and mind. Mostly the exercises are performed whilst sitting, the *Lotus Posture* being the recommended posture. Most modern people find it difficult to remain in this position, because their legs are too stiff, but with some months of practice you will be able to maintain the position. Remember that a posture should never become painful, and pay particular attention to your

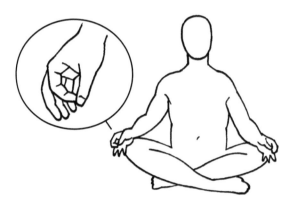

Cross-legged

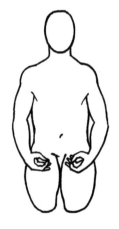

Diamond Posture

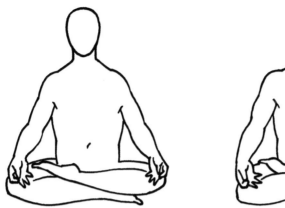

Half Lotus Posture

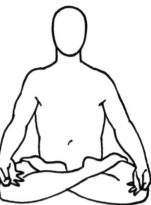

Lotus Posture

knees! When I practiced the *Lotus Posture* in the beginning, I sat in the position for only a few seconds, and increased later to a few minutes. When the legs are locked in the *Lotus Posture*, blood flow is inhibited to such an extent that your feet will become numb or may feel prickly. In the beginning your legs will become bluish, then grayish and marbled, but in time your legs and circulatory system will adapt to the posture, and you will be able to remain in the position effortlessly for a long time. When you want to get "out" of the position, move slowly and with control. It will often be quite difficult to stretch your legs completely, and it will be impossible to stand on them right away. Rub your legs with your hands and give them a minute's rest.

Other excellent postures and somewhat easier to perform are the *Half Lotus* and the *Diamond Posture*. If you cannot manage any of them, it will suffice to sit *Cross-legged* or sit on the front part of an even chair. Just remember to keep a straight back, the chest open and the abdomen relaxed. It is preferable, however, to attain a proper yoga posture since this will press key points (chakras), such as the genital region, which will aid in regulating prana. In addition, the amount of blood in your legs will be reduced and the surplus blood can then be directed to the heart, lungs and brain.

When you sit in *Cross-legged*, you have a large surface contact with the floor and thus have the greatest possible balance in the body. Finally, to sit "locked" on the floor provides some safety especially when you perform advanced exercises where the body may shake.

Some simple ground principles exist in pranayama that are advisable to follow:

1) Breathe as calmly and harmoniously as possible
2) Always inhale through the nose and make a little pre-tension in the abdomen
3) Keep your eyes shut and listen to your breath
4) Maintain your body in a natural position
5) Relax the muscles that are not in use (particularly face, neck and shoulders)
6) See that there is fresh air and an appropriate room temperature
7) Practice the same place and time each day and wear loose-fitting clothes
8) Remember your inner (possibly outer) smile
9) Practice three to six hours after a main meal
10) Never exceed your natural capacity

Pranayama can be beneficial to all, but it is important that you do not act prematurely. Remember that pranayama is a considerably delicate discipline. Hence, progress slowly and systematically because affecting your lungs, circulatory system and nervous system is a serious matter.

Do not expect to acquire a good shape or an unbreakable health by breathing in a certain way for just two minutes a day. More is needed. But on the other hand if you make an effort, you will experience positive changes. You may experience some positive changes straight away, but allow for a period of one to three months before the changes become permanent. To practice five to ten minutes of pranayama daily is a good beginning, and the three most important conditions to bear in mind will be time, patience and determination. As my Indian friend Umesh so aptly put it: "Slowly is better".

Relaxing pranayama

Let us consider two exercises that have a soothing effect on body and mind, because they influence the parasympathetic part of your nervous system (rest and digest). People suffering enhanced blood pressure, epilepsy, asthma, headaches, sleep deprivation, stress or depression can benefit from these exercises.

VICTORIOUS BREATH (UJJAYI)

Ujjayi means "victorious breath" which refers to the breath conquering restlessness and stress. It is often called "the psychic breath", because it has such an enormous impact on your mental condition. The word may also mean "warrior", and in this connection it refers to an expanding chest of a strong and proud warrior. In a figurative sense, *Victorious Breath* can be understood as conquering your inner demons: laziness, bad habits, fear etc. *Victorious Breath* is a fundamental part of every advanced pranayama exercise, and in my opinion the most important of them all.

The exercise is extremely simple: When you inhale, make a little constriction in your throat to produce an even hissing sound. I believe you can describe the sound as being a bit "dry" - almost like a whisper. If you say "ngg" when you inhale, I am quite sure that you are on track. The entire sound is somewhat like "nggeeeeeeeh". Try bringing your breath to a halt several times during the same breath – that is says "ngg", "ngg", "ngg" – then you will soon sense which part of the throat to move. Remember to keep the rest of your head and face completely relaxed. When you exhale, you can produce the sound "uee". The entire sound is "uee – hhhhh". When you learn to control where and how to constrict the throat, you can leave out the "ngg" and "uee" and just let the breath flow to the sounds of "eeeeeeehhh" during inhalation and "hhhhhhh-heee" during exhalation.

The sound you are hearing is an amplified version of the sound that occurs naturally when you breathe. According to the ancient scriptures, this sound is a kind of repeating prayer – a mantra that sounds like "so-ham". The key to *Victorious Breath* is the slight constriction in the throat, since this enables you to completely control the flow of air. By varying the degree of constriction in the throat, you can determine the amount of air that enters (or exits) and its velocity. It is the key to your perfect breath, and no other exercise is higher, stronger or more effective than *Victorious Breath*. You can perform it anywhere, standing, walking, lying down, running or swimming. Apart from the altogether calming effect, *Victorious Breath* is also useful to people who suffer stress, depression and asthma. *Victorious Breath* is applied to all asanas and as a fundamental element of many other pranayama exercises.

ALTERNATE NOSTRIL BREATHING (NADI SHODAN)

Nadi shodan means "purification of channels" and is an exercise used to clean your many energy channels (nadis). In *Alternate Nostril Breathing* you inhale through one nostril and exhale through the other to make the air flow in and out in a large upturned V. Recall that the cool moon flows in your left nostril (ida) and the warm sun flows in your right nostril (pingala). The purpose is to create a balance in your breath and thus your mental condition.

Sit in a comfortable position and place your right hand in front of you. Bend your index and middle finger to the palm of your hand. Move your hand up to below your nose. Now your thumb can shut the right nostril and your third finger, supported by the little finger, can shut the left nostril. Take care not to touch the skin with your nails, but only your fingertips. Alternatively, let the hand remain open and place your index and middle finger between your eyebrows. This will provide them with a good support, and it creates a distance that is appropriate for the fingers that will be shutting off the nostrils. Be careful not to create tensions in your shoulders or anywhere else in the body. Always use the right hand, even if you are left-handed.

Perform the exercise like this: Exhale through both nostrils. Shut the right nostril and inhale through the left nostril. Open the right nostril and shut the left while you exhale through the right nostril. Keep the left nostril shut and inhale through the right nostril. Open the left nostril, close the right and exhale through the left nostril. This constitutes one cycle. You will quickly sense the flow of air forming a large upturned V.

Feel free to combine this exercise with *Victorious Breath*. Aim at producing an inhalation and exhalation that are equally long. If you close your eyes, it is easier to sense what happens in your body. Try to direct the air as high up in the nose as possible and sense it there. You can also visualize the air flow e.g. as a gently flowing golden wave. If you would like to know what your breath looks like, place a little mirror below your nostrils and exhale. Then you will be able to see the flow of air. If you stand in front of a large mirror and place a little mirror below your nose, the flow will be even more visible - especially if you blow hard. It will look like the heat waves on asphalt on a hot summers day, and will resemble a little blazing fire.

Use ujjayi pranayama in the following table (breathe through both nostrils with a small constriction in the throat) or use alternate nostril breathing (alternate between shutting the right and left nostril) – with or without *Victorious Breath*.

The seconds indicated in the diagram are consultative and can be of longer or shorter duration or be exchanged with e.g. number of heart beats. Most important is the ratio inhalation: breath hold: exhalation: breath hold, that has to follow the table.

Since breath holding with full lungs (antara kumbhaka) and particularly with empty lungs (bahya kumbhaka) is part of the exercise, it is important to progress cautiously and patiently. When to proceed to the next level is indicated but can vary from person to person. You may be able to advance through the first levels within a matter of days. However, it may require months to reach the last level.

Each level is performed a minimum of 10 times in a row and preferably daily. Remember that you are not to become short of breath or gasp for breath – this is an indication that you have proceeded too quickly.

Pranayama

	Inhalation	Breath holding (full lungs)	Exhalation	Breath holding (empty lungs)	Ratio
1. week/ month	4 seconds	-------	8 seconds	-------	1:0:2:0
2. week/ month	4 seconds	4 seconds	8 seconds	-------	1:1:2:0
3. week/ month	4 seconds	4 seconds	8 seconds	4 seconds	1:1:2:1
4. week/ month	4 seconds	8 seconds	8 seconds	4 seconds	1:2:2:1
5. week/ month	4 seconds	8 seconds	8 seconds	8 seconds	1:2:2:2

Vitalizing pranayama

Pranayama does not only consist of slow and deep breaths aimed at soothing everything. Several of the exercises are relatively intense and refreshing, because they stimulate the sympathetic part of the nervous system that also increases heart frequency. Thus people suffering enhanced blood pressure, weak heart, epilepsy or reduced liver function have to be cautious when performing these exercises, or perform them relatively calmly. The exercises have a cleansing effect on the blood and develop the lungs, heart, circulatory system and particularly the diaphragm. Even better than a long swim or a marathon! They also clean the nose and sinuses and are therefore excellent at preventing colds and other more serious illnesses. In addition, they constitute a formidable alternative to nose flushing (neti) that is recommended prior to every training session. As something quite remarkable, the exercises are a kind of brain massage with the rapid breaths making the brain gently rock to and fro, because the blood pressure constantly changes. Breathing faster than usual directs excess oxygen to the body and brain. These pranayama exercises are thus very vitalizing.

Two of the most prevalent exercises that are performed in a sitting yoga posture are described below.

BRAIN PURIFICATION (KAPALABHATI)

Kapala means bowl, shell or skull and *bhati* shinning. Thus *kapalabhati* provides you with a shining, clean and clear head.

Sit on the floor with your hands along your sides or in your lap and empty your lungs more than usual. Now draw as much air into your lungs as possible – that is a long and deep inhalation. Blow the air out of your lungs in one fast blow by using your "stomach", like when you blow your nose, just faster. Release the tension in the abdominal muscles and diaphragm and let air passively flow in. Make sure that the stomach moves inwards and upwards and not outwards, when you exhale. This point is vital and a common beginner's mistake.

Begin with 10-15 repetitions, and with a little practice you will soon become strong enough to do more. When you can do 60-120 repetitions per minute, you have reached a satisfactory capacity, but it may take you months or even years. You can perform *Victorious Breath* during the exercise, but it has to be extremely weak. Remember that the chest has to remain passive during this exercise: only use the abdominal muscles and the diaphragm. This exercise works opposite to your usual breathing, because the inhalation is passive and the exhalation is active. The exercise strengthens brain function, memory and willpower.

BELLOWS BREATHING (BHASTRIKA)

Bhastrika means "bellow" and is in many ways similar to the brain purification exercise. However, the exercise is even more powerful and the air flow is created by the abdominal muscles, the diaphragm and the muscles in the chest. The stomach, intestines, visceral organs and especially the lungs are cleansed and strengthened. Empty your lungs while performing *Victorious Breath* and then draw a fast and deep inhalation (without *Victorious Breath*). Use your diaphragm when you exhale and do it quickly and forcefully, making sure your stomach moves inwards and upwards and not outwards. As mentioned above, this is of utmost importance. Inhalation as well as exhalation should be active and equally powerful. Begin with 10-15 breaths. A final goal would be 60 breaths per minute. To make the breathing even more forceful, you can use your arms and hands. Stretch your arms above your head, and move them down quickly while bending your elbows on the exhalation, clenching your fists at the same time. When you inhale, quickly return your arms to the stretched position and open your hands. You will quite easily feel the effect on the arms, exactly as if you were a living bellows. Like *Brain Purification* this exercise is a powerful hyperventilation where the carbon dioxide concentration in the body drops below its normal level. Be careful not to proceed too hastily, since it can lead to dizziness and even make you pass out briefly. Though, this is by no means dangerous and you will soon "wake up", often with a prickly sensation in the body that is not uncomfortable.

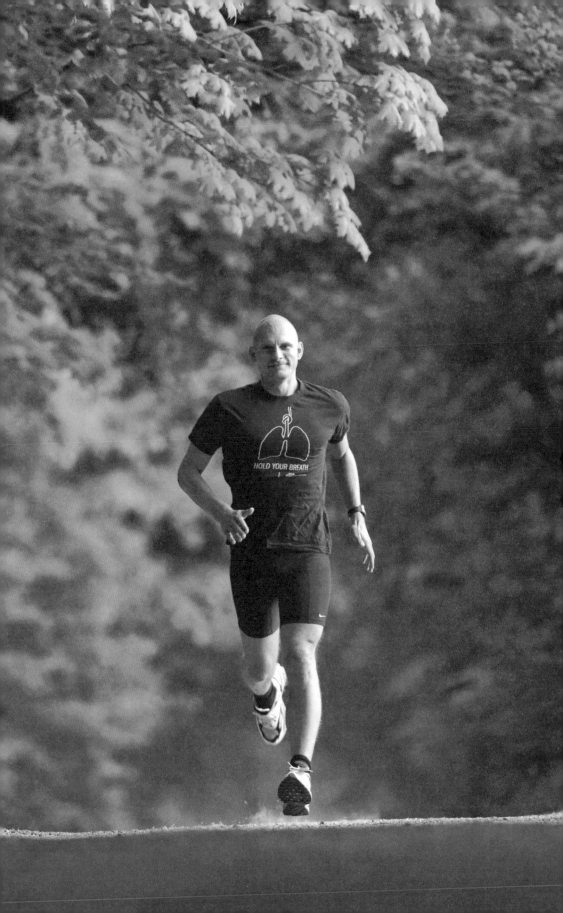

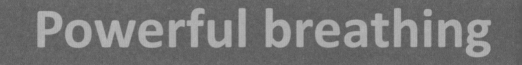

Powerful breathing

Optimize your athletic performance

The breath of sport

I hope that you by now have a sense of the positive effects of a relaxed body and a controlled breath. When you breathe efficiently, your body is cleansed of unwanted waste products, your lungs are strengthened and your nervous system is harmonized. Your thoughts calm down which enables you to control your stress level, lower your pulse and acquire more energy. You can do this in your everyday life, both at home and at work.

> "Those who breathe half, live half."
> ACHARYA MILIND KUMAR BHARDWAY

Now that you have acquired knowledge of the composition and function of the breath and have tried the first breathing and breath holding exercises, there are some obvious fields where you can start converting theory to practice. One of these fields is sports, and whether you practice sport occasionally or are an elite performer, the yoga and freediving techniques are bound to improve your results. In addition, they will make your training more thrilling, challenging, and not least, varied.

The breath is an integrated part of any type of sport and is adjusted according to needs. Naturally, the degree to which the breath is used varies and the span between a marathon runner and an archer is enormous. Scientifically and intuitively the breath is undoubtedly significant in reaching sports goals. Efficient breathing oxygenates all muscles of the body to make them work optimally and at the same time removes the carbon dioxide produced by every cell, in vast amounts, during activity. It is surprising how little attention the breath and all its facets are given in sports training, teaching and education. This may be because our Western culture has no tradition of considering something as diffuse and "airy" as the breath.

Muscles, however, are easy to relate to and athletes spend plenty of resources on improving and strengthening these. Even though muscles are the body's "engine", there are some limitations to training the muscles. For example, muscles are very heavy and a weight gain is not desirable to a rower, a horseman or a long distance runner.

"Citius, Altius, Fortius."
THE OLYMPIC MOTTO

In addition, larger muscles enhance oxygen and sugar consumption which would be catastrophic to a freediver or long distance swimmer. An elite athlete, whose muscles are trimmed and trained to his or her particular sport, is not able to improve performance by brute strength. A simple yet overlooked solution is to reduce the mass of muscle slightly, but at the same time increase the supply of oxygen to each cell, so that the overall capacity is not reduced. It is only body weight and the gross energy consumption that is reduced.

By working with the breath it is possible to improve performance, and this is exactly why there is a lot to be gained from training the lungs, especially if we consider them as the "filter" and "tank" of the body. If at the same time you enhance the quality of the air that reaches the lungs (higher "octane"), the body will be able to increase performance in the short as well as the long term, becoming more explosive and capable of sustained effort. A conscious and well-adjusted breath also provides the means to complete mental control which every athlete desires – particularly in stressed situations.

"In order to keep in shape I run, play tennis, squash, swim and ride my bicycle. In particular when I run and ride my bicycle, I use my breath to settle into a rhythm and also to enhance my capacity. During the first 10-15 minutes of my training sessions, I am focused on creating a rhythm in my movement and breath to give myself the best premises for a long performance. When some time has elapsed and I do interval training, I try to expand my capacity by varying the seconds I inhale versus exhale. In this way I gain a greater control of my breath during the exercise which again enhances my performance on shorter and longer distances."

Heidi Have, 38
Corporate Account Manager, Hewlett-Packard

There is no doubt that in most sports changing one's mental aspects can quickly improve an athlete. Sports psychology is thus extremely interesting to work with. But before you shape the mental layers of an athlete, it is essential that the "engine" is well-lubricated and equipped with the most horsepowers possible.

Therefore, let us take a closer look at where breathing and breath holding can optimize different physiological processes. Some of the ideas I present below may seem a bit far-fetched compared to your daily training. However, below is a set of concrete examples that I hope can adequately support this idea.

Good lungs

It is not surprising that athletes in good condition as well as singers and musicians that play wind instruments often have a larger lung volume than average. The elasticity of the lungs and the ability to contract them are important elements of the breathing process.

The elasticity of the lungs and chest is particularly important, because it expresses the normal resistance the lungs face during the active part of the breath, the inhalation. The more elastic, the less energy is required to fill the lungs: as you obviously breathe quite frequently, and often forcefully, there is much energy to save here.

Practice breathing exercises to strengthen the muscles involved and give them more endurance. Perform stretching exercises to soften the muscles and tendons in the chest. This will, in a matter of weeks, develop effective and harmonious breathing.

In freediving many of these stretching exercises are performed with the lungs completely full – as opposed to in other sports. However, some techniques are necessary. A useful one to enhance your lung volume above your normal maximal capacity is by "lung packing" which is widely used in freediving but requires alertness. Never pack too much air in your lungs at once and remember to listen to your body as you progress – preferably guided by an instructor.

An experiment performed on Swedish elite swimmers showed that five to six weeks of practicing packing can significantly enhance one's lung capacity. This is important because a greater lung volume results in more oxygen in each breath and an improved excretion of carbon dioxide. In addition, a greater lung volume improves the buoyancy making the swimmer able to float higher in the water, resulting in less water resistance. A larger lung volume also results in more oxygen to all the cells, providing a faster recovery of the body after the periods of intense work that are part of sports like handball, football and ice hockey.

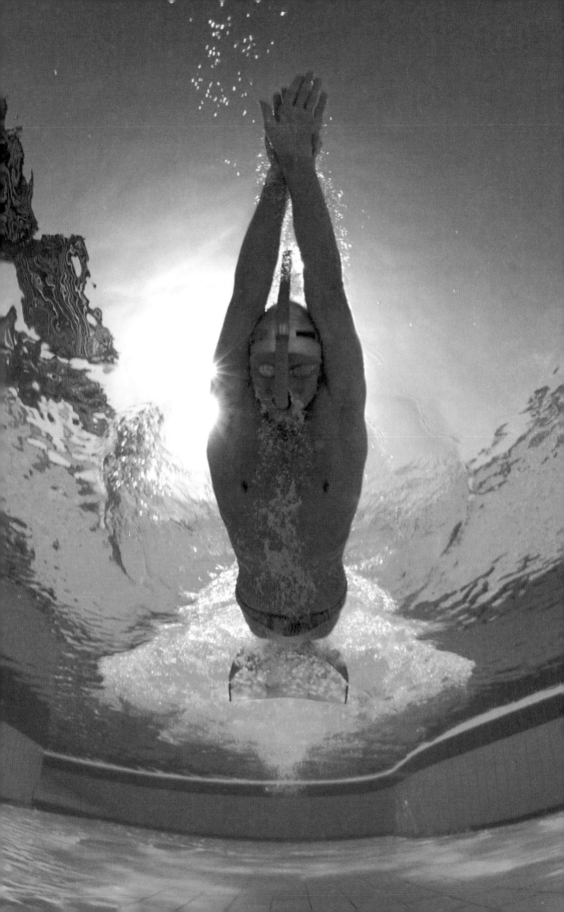

If inhaling through the nose and exhaling through the mouth is employed during a break, an optimal effect is achieved. This is due to a small gas molecule *nitrogen oxide* (NO) in the nasal cavity that enhances the oxygenation of blood in the lungs during inhalation while carbon dioxide most readily escapes through the mouth during exhalation.

> "Stig has been helping out coaching my swimmers to optimize their breathing which is crucial to an elite swimmer. He has demonstrated that yoga and breathing exercises can increase lung capacity."
>
> Bo Jacobsen, 43, head coach of WestSwim Esbjerg
> 4 times world champion and former world record holder in fin swimming

Another interesting phenomenon of the lungs is that they show variation during the day, like the nose. There are periods where the lungs work better. A detail such as this and a small percentage of increased lung volume may seem trivial to some, but to many, such as elite athletes and devoted everyday athletes, it is a matter of optimizing performance and to get all you can out of it. Pennies make dollars.

Heart and blood

Athletes that train cardiovascular disciplines often have large hearts and a highly branched vascular system. With powerful breathing exercises you can obtain the same cardiovascular training efficiently and quickly. If an athlete is prevented from exercising, these are wonderful alternative exercises to perform. Countless possibilities exist to keep fit through breathing even during a prolonged injury that impedes normal movement. Even breath holding is an interesting alternative, since it stimulates the heart as well as the circulatory system.

Efficient breathing possesses a unique ability to influence blood circulation as well as its composition and acidity. As previously described, the diving reflex is triggered by breath holding as well as contact with water. Whereupon, the spleen contracts and releases its store of red blood cells to the body, thereby increasing the oxygen reserve of the blood. I can image several sports where this would provide an enormous advantage. If you hold your breath on empty or near empty lungs, the effect would be even greater and occur faster.

Swimming training strengthens lung capacity because the natural resistance of water exercises all the respiratory muscles.

Usually very fit athletes do not have a large fraction of red blood cells in their blood (hematocrit value) but instead a large amount of blood. If blood becomes too "thick", it simply cannot move through all the fine blood vessels fast enough. However, it would be interesting to investigate how a brief rise in the number of red blood cells could affect a sports performance.

Different breath holding exercises influence the blood on a long-term basis by stimulating the natural hormone *EPO* (erythropoietin) in the kidneys. This hormone promotes the formation of red blood cells in our bone marrow where approximately 2-3 million are produced each second. However, an equal amount is broken down by the kidney each second.

Thus breath holding is a practical and cheap solution to enhance the content of red blood cells in the blood as compared to high altitude training or spending time in an altitude simulation tent (hypoxic tent), which has the same effect.

Muscles and brain

More oxygen in the muscle cells will naturally enhance performance and enable them to work harder and for a longer stretch of time before they acidify. When you breathe vigorously (hyperventilate), it is possible to remove a large amount of carbon dioxide from the blood, and make it more alkaline. Experiments have shown that muscles performing moderate work perform better in alkaline conditions.

Another important element in the muscles is the oxygen binding protein, myoglobin, which is related to blood hemoglobin. However, myoglobin is less willing to release oxygen, and is thus an extra reserve of oxygen in the muscle cells. As opposed to the amount of hemoglobin that can be affected, it is difficult to alter the amount of myoglobin in the muscles.

A hypothesis suggests that prolonged low oxygen tension in the muscles can affect the amount of myoglobin. This state could be achieved by activating the diving reflex and diving with empty lungs in very cold water (without a wetsuit). It is extreme, but nevertheless interesting, because an increased amount of myoglobin does not only result in more oxygen to the muscles, but also a higher buffer capacity for various waste products in the cell and with it a delay in the production of lactic acid. This is what seals and whales do, and it works!

In order to affect the nervous system and in particular the brain, a strong diving reflex is of great importance. We have observed how breath holding can make the pulse drop rapidly, and this is obviously advantageous in many sports. The immediate result is an enhanced focus and calmness.

Another method that can be readily employed is to cover your face, especially the forehead and the area around the nose, with a cold wet towel. The *trigeminal nerve* is situated in this area, which will initiate the diving reflex by lowering the pulse and relaxing the body. In this way you can quickly calm your nerves before a match. By training your diving response, it is possible to modify the signal to the brain that carbon dioxide level is high. After a prolonged breath hold, people will usually have the urge to breathe, because the level of carbon dioxide is high - not because the oxygen level is low. In other words, the body is able to continue the breath hold. In well-trained freedivers the nervous system is adapted to tolerate high carbon dioxide levels, and breathing is only initiated when the oxygen level reaches a critical minimum.

An experiment with a group of triathlon athletes showed that three weeks of breath holding exercises was enough to increase carbon dioxide tolerance significantly. Naturally, this is relevant to all sports because it means that an athlete can push him or herself further. The deep

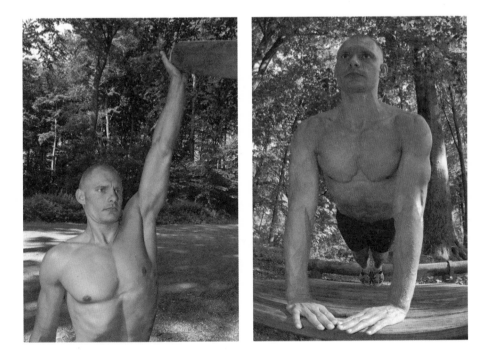

harmonious breath is also worth considering, since by way of the vagus nerve it immediately makes the body relax. Particularly effective is a slow exhalation where you make a sound by creating a little air resistance with the lips "psssss" – try it yourself!

The mental breath

Where the physical abilities come short, the mental part takes over. Employing mental tools can move yourself or another human much further and faster than it is possible by physical and technical means alone. In all modesty, I believe that one of my greatest forces is the ability to believe in dreams on the behalf of other people - in many cases, long before they imagine them on their own. Whether this belief is due to my naivety or childish super optimism, I will leave to others to decide.

During the Freediving World Championship in Japan 2010, I coached the Danish National team. In the line up the reigning French world champions presented a very strong team as did nations such as New Zealand, Japan and Finland – in other words, the Danish team were the underdogs.

The three Danish athletes were in excellent physical shape and had prepared themselves in the best possible manner before the championship. However, they were all quite inexperienced with competitions at high level. Thus, my biggest challenge was to convince them that they were ready to perform the best dives of their lives by pushing beyond their present limits. Amazingly, they all managed to control the high stress load and went way beyond their personal bests.

I achieved this by applying imagery techniques to strengthen their mental anchors and belief in their own abilities. The key challenge was to impose the best possible psychological approach for the individual athlete. I convinced their subconscious minds to achieve this incredible performance by presenting them specific aims and explaining them in detail how and why they were ready to realize these goals.

In the finals they fulfilled their dream of becoming the new world champions by pushing their body, mind and soul way beyond their comfort zone. These beautiful and controlled dives earned them the Free-diving World Championship 2010. I am thrilled to have been part of this amazing achievement and I am extremely proud of our ability to work as a team.

Modern sports psychology focuses on mental training, where an athlete tries to strengthen his or her psychological profile by modification of attitudes, objectives, motivation, performance anxiety, concentration

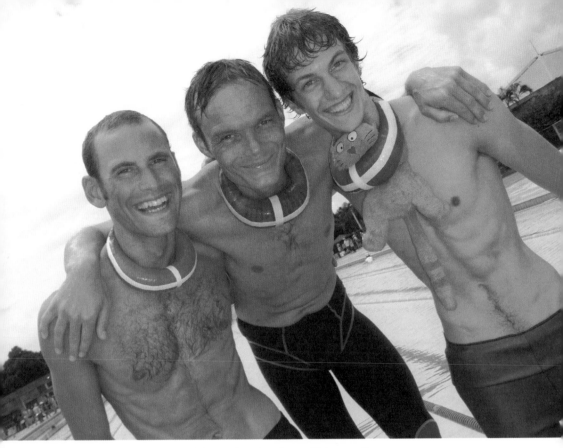

Nursing a strong team spirit can lead to incredible results.

etc. There is also an enormous focus on psychosomatic relaxation, visualization, autogenic training and a long list of other techniques.

These techniques are in many ways very useful, but they are primarily "thought techniques" and as such have weaknesses. In some instances you may not have the time or peace to practice them – either before or after a competition; and if the mind is running and tensions build in the body, they can result in a negative effect. For some, resignation or panic is close at hand.

The breath does not play a major role in modern sports psychology and is employed for relaxation rather than as a psychological tool. There are two main reasons why breathing is a strong and reliable mental tool. Firstly, to most it is always easier to control compared with thoughts, as long as you are conscious about it. Complete mental control can be achieved in a simple way, which is the basis of yoga and especially pranayama.

The second reason lies in "classical conditioning". About 100 years ago the Russian physiologist Ivan Pavlov made dogs salivate by the sound of a bell. He achieved this by ringing the bell each time the dogs received their meal. After some time the dogs associated the sound of the bell with food, and thus began to salivate as soon as they heard the bell, even though there was no food in front of them.

In the same way I believe that the mind can be "conditioned" by the breath and this is not only restricted to the world of sports. When a positive, focused or relaxed mood is linked to the breath, it will be a great resource if the mind or "nerves" fail. You have created a new mental anchor. The breath directly influences the body, whereas e.g. imagery focuses on a particular part of the brain. Because the breath is dynamic and alive, it influences body and mind at the same time. This will create a positive feedback and ping-pong effect, resulting in a bright and controlled mind along with a well-balanced and strong body.

When the connection between the breath and a special mental state has grown strong, it will relieve the mental processes by acting as a "trigger". In other words, a particular breath will in itself be enough to achieve a desired focused state, leaving more of the brain's resources available.

There are many other benefits hidden in the breath, particularly because its rhythm is so closely tied to the movements of the body. By becoming more aware of the finer nuances of the breath, the body's performance can be optimized. You can be relaxed at the right moment, but tense or rigid a moment later. Many athletes already work with such techniques but often on a subconscious level. Through an increased focus on the breath, physical awareness is also sharpened.

Because the breath is a firm focus point, it may also be used to distract. It can be a great help especially in association with pain or even when you are just exhausted or submitted to mental stress (e.g. during a penalty kick or field goal).

Finally, I believe that the breath can be a shortcut to achieving a state of flow. This phenomenon consists of the fusion of the body and mind, where time ceases and things happen by themselves. This often occurs in sports and can contribute to achieving exceptional results. This state of comfort also occurs during breath holds, often surprisingly fast.

With a holistic approach to the significance of the breath, a greater effect can be achieved on the conscious as well as the subconscious level. This is the unique power of the breath.

Breathing experiments

The more we learn about the breath and its connection to the body and mind, the better we can apply the various breathing and breath holding techniques to sports and the treatment of illnesses.

Physicians, biologist and scientists find freedivers worth studying, because we can hold our breath for such a long time under controlled conditions. In this way, it is possible to examine how different organs react to extreme conditions, such as when the body is subject to a low oxygen tension (hypoxia) and is forced to function differently or in a new way. Persons that suffer chronic illnesses or have been subject to an acute accident may experience similar extreme conditions in the body, but they cannot be analyzed in a controlled fashion.

Studying freedivers is particularly relevant, because they provide scientists with useful knowledge that can be used to create better treatments and therapies. This knowledge can benefit people suffering heart failures, cerebral thrombosis or damage to parts of the nervous system. Of course, this knowledge is more widely applicable to scientific work, but freedivers can profit from the information by using it to establish new training methods as well.

I have participated in many scientific studies through the years, often as a "guinea pig". It has been exciting, rewarding and very interesting to participate in these pioneering studies that have been concerned with the breath and notably breath holding on land and in water. The organs that scientists have been targeting in the studies have been the heart, brain and lungs, since these are of the greatest significance to the health of the body and its performance under stress.

The strong heart

My heart has been examined in different places over the world. Once by the physicians Rubén Leta and Francesc Carreras, from Barcelona, who performed an ultrasound scanning of my heart. In such a scanning you can observe whether the different heart chambers are being filled with blood as they should, and you can evaluate whether the heart valves open and close, when they should. My heart was normal and in a good shape. Possibly with a tendency to an enlarged left heart ventricle, which is observed in many athletes that practice sport on an elite level and is thus called an "athlete's heart".

During the study I held my breath for nearly seven minutes, which the physicians had not witnessed before, and towards the end my pulse dropped to about 30 beats per minute, which is approximately 10 beats below my normal resting pulse. Try registering your own pulse – place your finger on the carotid artery for a minute and count.

On another occasion my heart was scanned at Skejby Hospital in Aarhus, Denmark, by the heart specialist, Anders Kirstein. Again, I held my breath for more than seven minutes and achieved an even lower pulse. I stressed myself a bit, but the Doctor acted "cool" during the investigation, even when my face turned from purple to colorless, and the pulse became very difficult to register! Moreover, a television crew was doing a feature on the experiment, which made the situation even more intense.

I later visited Labman Hawaii Inc. and the heart specialist, Neal Shikuma. For the first time I produced a flat line on a heart monitor - that is, my heart did not beat for four to five seconds. In order to do this, I used an advanced technique known in freediving and yoga, and according to Doctor Shikuma, a pause in the heart beats of a normal heart such as this had never been registered at his clinic before. My heart was healthy and normal, but Doctor Shikuma expressed concern as to whether it was a good idea to continue training on an elite level, because it might lead to heart illnesses.

It is quite obvious that you should not practice any kind of sport at high intensity without recovering or taking actual breaks off from training, but I must admit that I was not particularly worried. At that time my heart appeared normal and felt and worked fabulously. This was also confirmed by the Italian heart specialist Alessandro Pingitore and his team of scientists that examined a number of top freedivers during a World Championship in deep diving.

Since then, I have asked him to examine the observations that were done on my heart thoroughly, and Doctor Pingitore has confirmed that my heart seems healthy and in good shape. The study actually showed that the freediver's heart works better than normal after a deep dive. This could possibly be caused by the diving reflex directing more blood to the lungs during and after the dive. Nonetheless, I find this observation intriguing. It seems that freediving can make the heart more relaxed and function better at the same time.

Normal oxygenated blood is red, whereas blood after a seven-minute breath hold is very dark because of the low oxygen content.

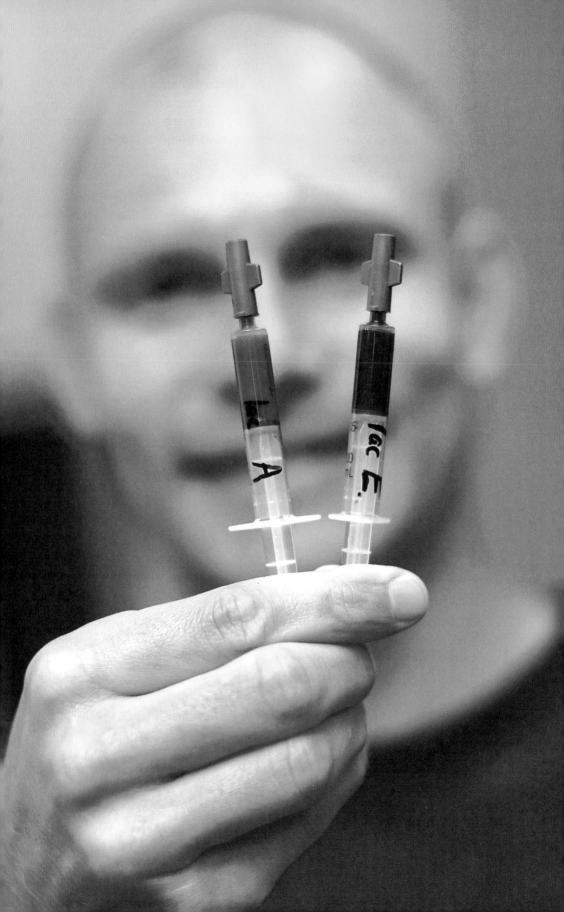

Another investigation was conducted by the French doctor, Frédéric Lemaître, during a large international competition in Monaco, where the world's best freedivers were invited to compete in the discipline Static Apnea (breath holding). For the first time, this study established that elite freedivers differed from other good freedivers in realizing a secondary pulse drop during the dive.

Popularly speaking, elite freedivers have an extra "low gear" that they can employ when it becomes necessary. Naturally, this economizes oxygen consumption and extends breath holding. Whether this "gear" is inborn or actualized through hard and determined training is yet to be discovered. I must admit that I believe the latter is true, as another example of the fantastic ability of the human body to adapt to new circumstances.

The sublime brain

Besides my heart, my brain has also been subject to scans. The objective of these experiments has been to achieve a greater understanding of how the brain reacts when oxygen supplies decrease. These experiments aim to lead to new or supplementary treatments in cases of strokes in the brain (cerebral thrombosis or hemorrhages).

The ultrasound scanning enables the scientists to take a look inside the brain and get an impression of how different areas of the brain look, how great the blood flow is, how much oxygen is consumed in the various parts of brain tissue, and a number of other activities.

My first brain scan was performed by Doctor Christine Sølling, who worked on cerebral thrombosis at the time. For two days I held my breath for approximately seven minutes while my brain was scanned.

One of the nurses believed there was something wrong with the last blood sample because it was almost black or the color of a very dark red wine, naturally caused by low oxygen content. On the other hand, when blood is completely oxygenated it is very red. Even though my blood had low oxygen content at the end of the experiment, there were no signs of damage to the brain tissue. Neither on a short-term, nor on a long-term basis.

Doctor Mahmoud Ashkanian later performed a new brain scan to investigate the influence of carbogen on the oxygen uptake of the brain. Carbogen is a mixture of carbon dioxide and oxygen, in this case 5% carbon dioxide and 95% oxygen. The idea of using this mixture of gas as a treatment came from cancer therapy. It has been shown that certain kinds of cancer are more sensitive to radiation therapy if the tissue is well oxygenated, and carbogen has the capacity to improve the extent of oxygenation of the tissue.

There are two main reasons why it is advantageous to employ carbogen. As previously described, oxygen is a life necessity to the survival of every cell, but only in the right concentration. If you are subject to pure oxygen for a long stretch of time it acts as a deadly poison. Oxygen also has the ability to constrict the blood vessels. Thus, if you suffer cerebral thrombosis, it is not appropriate to treat with pure oxygen, which we actually do at the moment. In ambulances, swimming pools etc. the life-saving equipment contains pure oxygen.

Carbon dioxide has the opposite effect since it creates dilation of the blood vessels. As you may recall, carbon dioxide is a waste product that is produced in the cells when they work. Nevertheless, carbon dioxide should not be considered a pure waste product that has to be eliminated immediately, because it has a positive effect on the blood vessels, making them relax and expand. In addition, it is part of the regulation of the breathing cycle by continuously affecting the breathing center of the brain.

> "Over the oxygen supply of the body
> carbon dioxide spreads its protective wings."
> JOHAN FRIEDERICH MIESCHER, 1885

In 2005 my friend William Trubridge (World Champion in deep diving) from New Zealand wrote the following in an email where we discussed optimal breathing techniques prior to a deep dive: "Remember, CO_2 is your friend". It is worth considering that by regulating your breath you can manipulate the concentration of carbon dioxide in the blood and thus its acidity (pH). However, there are limits to how much carbon dioxide the body can tolerate.

The experiments with carbogen were successful and the results promising. The hypothesis is as follows: It will be beneficial to increase the amount of oxygen in the blood and at the same time direct more blood to the tissue which has been damaged, because the oxygen concentration of the tissue will rise. In this way you gain the beneficial effects of oxygen as well as carbon dioxide at the same time.

Another interesting observation resulted from the experiments. Several observations suggest that the brain – particularly two areas in the brain stem – appear different in freedivers compared to non-freedivers.

One area, the *Pons* (a structure on the brain stem), is involved in the regulation of the breathing process. The other area being the *Thalamus*, which functions as a relay station because it receives sensory inputs and determines which of these signals to forward to the cerebral cortex located in the cerebrum.

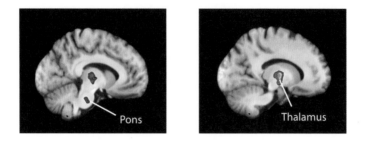

A freediver's brain is different from people who do not freedive - particularly in the areas of the brain stem shown on the brain scans.

The studies are yet preliminary and limited, but the results are compelling, because they indicate that different centers in the brain can likely be exercised and developed through breathing exercises – especially breath holding. This opens new perspectives in relation to training and not least, rehabilitation of people suffering brain damage.

In people who practice yoga and meditation, positive changes in the brain structure have been observed as well. Those most deeply involved in meditation show the greatest changes in brain structure. So scientific research is on the verge of proving that it can be beneficial to meditate and practice breath holds once in a while!

A new study with the Danish brain scientist Peter Vestergaard-Poulsen from Aarhus, has shown that various exercises (e.g. conscious breathing, concentration and mindfulness meditation) are associated with anatomical changes in the structure of the brain stem. Notably, one area in the brain stem shows a greater density of nerve cells. Remarkably, this area is related to the regulation of our breath and heart rhythm, and is the place where the vagus nerve stems from.

It is the first time scientists have demonstrated an indication of plasticity in the brain stem, which means that humans, by means of the breath and thought, may be able to change the structure of the brain. This is not surprising, when you think about how stress can destroy the brain. But solid scientific investigations are what we approve of in the West!

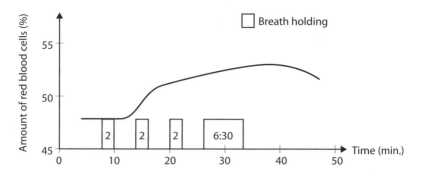

After a prolonged breath hold the amount of red blood cells increases because the spleen contracts.

Plenty of red blood cells

Another organ that is of interest to sports and the health services is the spleen, which works both as a destructive facility and a store of red blood cells. A couple of years ago my spleen was investigated by a Swedish Professor of Zoophysiology, Erika Schagatay, who for years has been a leading scientist in research into the diving response of man. On scans she could show how the spleen contracted during and after a prolonged breath hold. This knowledge is certainly useful since the spleen releases many red blood cells during contraction, thereby increasing the oxygen reserve of the body.

To be certain that the red blood cells did not originate from somewhere else in the body, people without a spleen were subject to the same conditions. This group did not show an elevation in the amount of red blood cells after prolonged breath holding which showed that the likely origin of the increase in red blood cells was the spleen.

Curiously, the size of my spleen seemed to pulse prior to the breath hold. To me, this suggests that the spleen could be under a mental influence and because I knew I was about to hold my breath it reacted. A psychological effect via the thought was created to influence the self-propelled autonomic nervous system.

One of the great secrets of yoga is its ability to gain control over the entire nervous system, also the part that usually cannot be controlled by will. A control such as this permeates deeper than modern science can imagine, but perhaps this is an indication of a psychosomatic phenomenon that can easily be tested in the future.

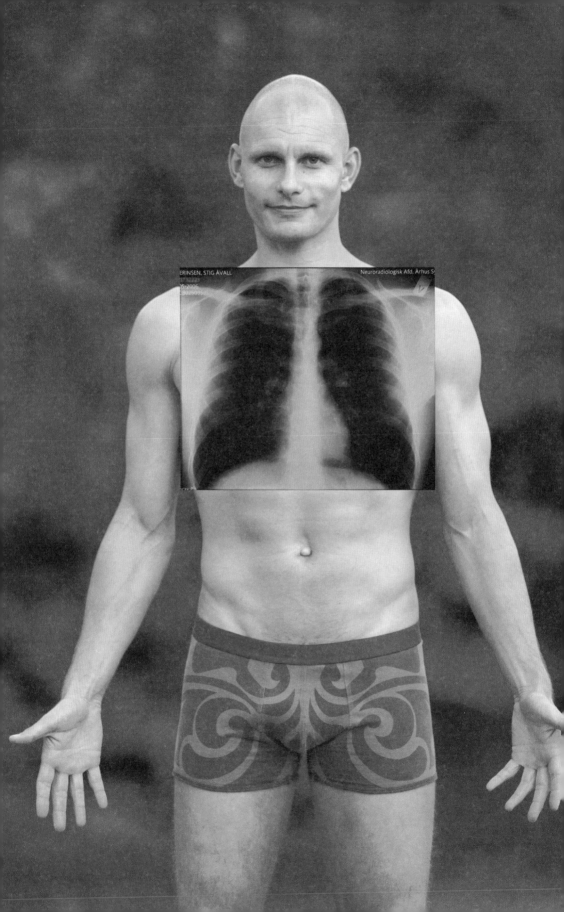

After more than six minutes breath holding, my spleen had shrunk to half its size (from 600 ml to 300 ml) and released a large amount of red blood cells to the blood stream at the same time. The increase in the amount of red blood cells was quite enormous, about 10%. This corresponds to an increase from 48% to 53% in the hematocrit value, which is the volume percentage of red blood cells in the blood. Your hematocrit value is probably around 42% to 45%. Men have a somewhat higher hematocrit value than women.

The notion that the blood's capacity to carry oxygen can be boosted by holding your breath is not only important to freedivers and other athletes, but certainly also to patients who need to strengthen the body's oxygen balance. Furthermore, this insight can be used as a healthy and ethical alternative to artificially produced EPO (erythropoietin) and other forbidden drugs. Naturally, this is most important in the case where a person cannot tolerate an injection of artificial EPO during treatment.

Recent studies have also shown that the correct breath hold training program can make the natural EPO concentration rise 24% in one day, which is immensely interesting when it comes to adding more red blood cells to the blood and thereby increase the oxygen level in a short time.

The lungs *can* be expanded permanently

The limit to the amount of air you can have in your lungs is usually higher than what people typically believe. It is relatively simple to measure how much the lungs are able to expand and thus the amount of extra air they can hold.

When you empty your lungs completely and then inhale as much air as you can, you obtain a measure of the total amount of air that the lungs contain. This is called the vital capacity (VC) and is typically four-five liters. The vital capacity is the amount of air that can be forced out after a maximal inhalation. It is the unit that is often referred to in connection with lung measurements.

After a normal exhalation a large amount of air still remains in the lungs and is called the functional residual capacity (FRC). If you then force as much air out as you possibly can by bending over and pressing your stomach and diaphragm, a small amount of air termed the residual volume (RV) will even still remain in the lungs.

The lungs can be expanded by training and the lower parts may extend well down along the back.

If you add the vital capacity to the residual volume (VC + RV) you get the total lung capacity (TLC), which is typically five-seven liters.

As previously mentioned, some freedivers employ a special air-packing method where the tongue is used as a piston. It is thus possible to pump even more air into the lungs thereby increasing total lung capacity. It is also possible to empty your lungs beyond the residual volume by reversing this technique (negative packing) after a maximal exhalation.

This technique has, to my knowledge, not been described anywhere, not even in the advanced yoga scriptures; nonetheless, negative packing is widely used in elite freediving. Particularly, to adapt the lungs and chest to the enormous pressure the body experiences during deep dives.

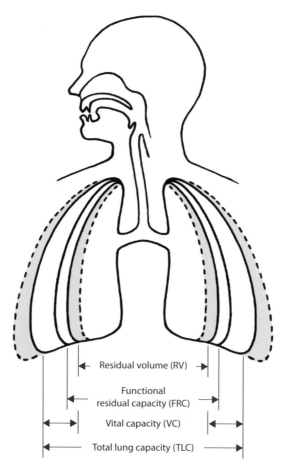

Different volumes of the lung and the effect of packing (outer blue area) and negative packing (inner blue area).

During a study at Aarhus University in Denmark, my total lung capacity was measured to more than 14 liters, which amounts to almost twice the capacity of the normal lungs of a person of the same height. This was obtained by packing almost three liters of air after a maximal inhalation. Packing leads to a larger amount of air and thus oxygen in the lungs. Put plainly, the battery of the body is enlarged. This enables you to hold your breath for a longer period of time, and packing has been employed in all freediving World Records within the last five years.

In addition, packing leads to a permanently enhanced lung volume. When the lungs and chest are compressed and expanded beyond the normal limits, the vital capacity is also enhanced which is significant to its performance and good health throughout life. There is now scientific evidence putting to rest the old myth that the volume of the lungs cannot be enhanced through training. However, it is extremely important to stress the fact that packing can potentially be dangerous. In the worst-case scenario, the lung membrane can burst because the pressure in the lungs is tripled. Therefore, packing should only be performed by experienced people or under professional supervision.

It is not difficult to see the vital significance of the breath to all the processes in the body. The examples above have described many effects that breathing and breath holds can have in optimizing sports performances. At the same time, similar breathing techniques can be used advantageously to prevent, or if the damage is already done, soothe or even cure patients during treatment. It is clear from the experiments that different breathing techniques have much to offer.

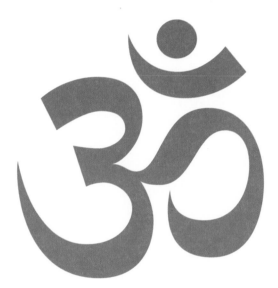

Exercises

In the following exercises are some simple but very efficient methods on how to strengthen and improve your breath and breath holds in your daily training. The following six exercises are excellent to warm-up with because they build and supple your entire body, particularly the chest. The first four exercises are performed standing and the last two while sitting.

1) CHEST AND SHOULDER STRETCH

Let your arms hang down along the side of your body and pull your shoulders back as far as possible during an inhalation. Maintain the pull for a couple of seconds and then cross your arms in front of the body while you exhale fully and let your chest relax. Repeat five-ten times in every direction.

Chest and shoulder stretch

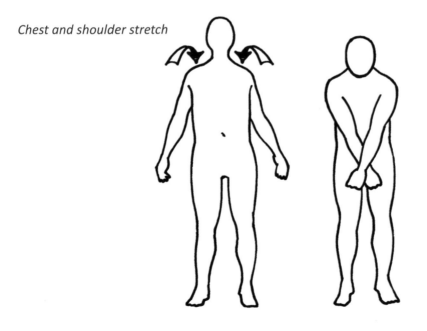

2) ALBATROS

Begin with a deep inhalation and stretch your arms above your head. After a brief pause exhale while the arms are lowered. Repeat 5-10 times. Perform the exercise calmly and match the breath to the movements.

Subsequently, begin with your arms in front of you (palms facing each other) and breathe in while the arms are pulled as far back as possible. Take a brief pause and move the arms to the front during exhalation. Repeat 5-10 times. Perform the exercise smoothly and match your breath to the movements.

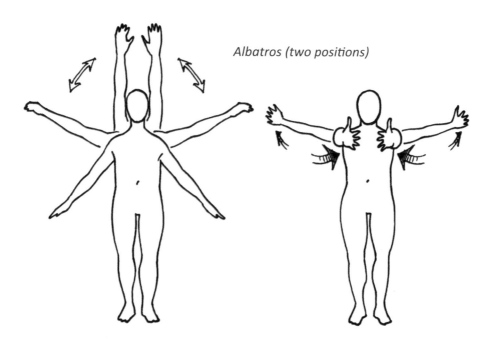

Albatros (two positions)

Repeat the two exercises above in a flowing, dynamic but fast movement 12-20 times. Perform the exercise using force and speed, but remember to match breath and movement.

3) SKY STRETCH

Stretch one arm up as far above your head as you can while you slowly breathe in. Maintain the stretch if possible (lungs full) for 5-10 seconds and exhale slowly. Now switch to the other arm. Repeat 10 times on each side. When the arm is lowered, exhale slowly and with control. If you can, stand on your toes to stretch the entire body.

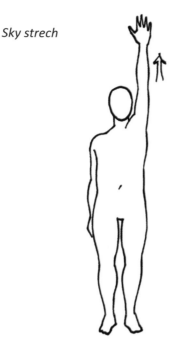

Sky strech

4) RAG DOLL

Bend over and angle your knees a bit. Let your arms dangle free on the ground. Breathe calmly and say "ahhhhh" during the exhalation. Let your body relax, particularly the neck, shoulders, jaw, cheeks, tongue and eyes.

Rag doll

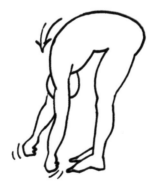

To achieve maximum strength, endurance and flexibility in your lungs and chest, I recommend two "Popeye"-exercises that can be performed with a *Victorious Breath*.

5) NATURAL CHEST PRESS (TARZAN)

Press hard against the sides of your rib cage with the palms of your hands during inhalation and exhalation. Check your breath constantly to see if you can squeeze the remaining air out of your lungs during exhalation. Hold your breath 5-10 seconds between each breath.

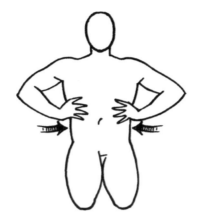

Tarzan

6) ARTIFICIAL CHEST PRESS (SNAKE)

Tie a bicycle tube or some other elastic material around your chest and inhale and exhale slowly and with control. Possibly hold your breath 5-10 seconds between each breath. If the tube is tied low around your chest, it will particularly strengthen the muscles of the abdomen and diaphragm.

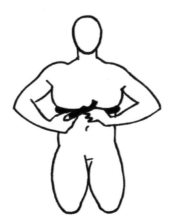

Snake

7) RHYTHM AND RATIO TRAINING

This kind of exercise is fun and easily applied to other kinds of exercises like walking, running, swimming, riding a bicycle, weight lifting or some other exercise. Whatever number you use of steps, breast strokes, repetitions or seconds, the point of this exercise is to apply a ratio to your inhalation, breath holding and exhalation.

If you are running you could try a 2:2:4 ratio – that is two steps to inhale, two steps to hold your breath and finally four steps to exhale.

You may also employ a 2:4:2, 2:4:8 etc. ratio – or try completely different combinations. Find your own rhythm where you do not get exhausted, and slowly increase from week to week.

The exercises practice breath control. They will make you breathe more easily and can change your body's tolerance to low oxygen and high carbon dioxide levels.

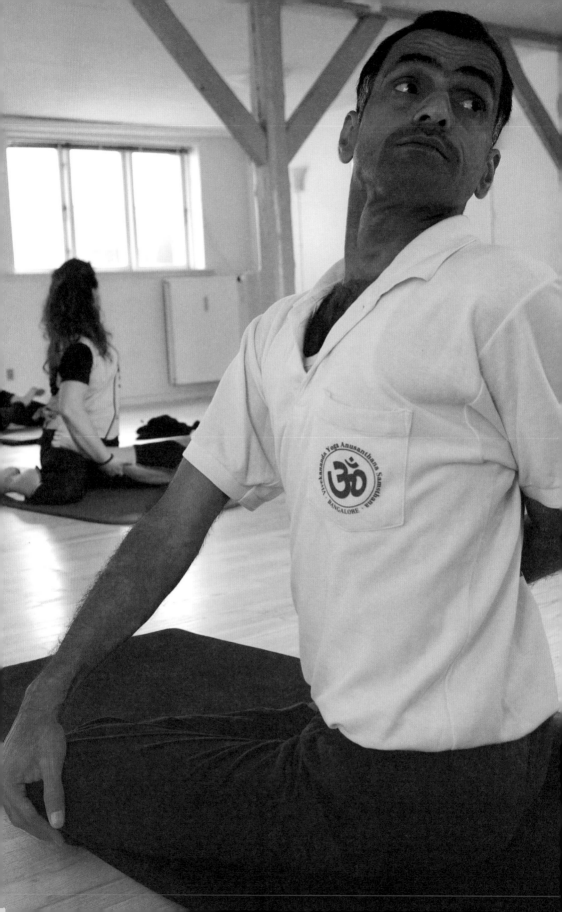

Therapeutic breathing

Get well faster

A long and healthy life

To a large extent our health is determined by how much we breathe and how we do it. Many illnesses could be avoided, if only we breathed properly. At first glance, the idea that your breath is tied to whether you have elevated blood pressure, pneumonia, depression, stress or even just a headache may seem a bit eccentric, but recall that your breath directly affects your circulatory system i.e. your lungs, heart, blood and lymph vessels, digestion, hormone production, nerves - even your thoughts and emotions. Viewed in this way, it is not difficult to understand that the best way to stay healthy is to care for your breathing – train it and be aware of how to make the best of it. If you do not care about your breath or misuse it, it can have severe consequences.

> "Those who fail to take the time to be healthy
> will ultimately have to take the time to be sick."
> JAMES CHAPPELL

This quote is supported by a large medical study called The Framingham Heart Study. This study was initiated in 1948 and based in Framingham, Massachusetts. More than 5,000 adult subjects from the City of Framingham were selected, and the study continues today with the third generation (the grandchildren of the original subjects) participa-ting. The main object has been to identify the factors that lead to cardiovascular diseases by monitoring subjects over a long-term study.

All of the subjects were given a thorough medical examination every other year (measuring blood pressure, blood sugar, cholesterol, pulse, lung volume etc.), their physical shape was determined and a lifestyle interview (diet and smoking habits, exercise etc.) was given along with the physical tests. The first set of conclusions appeared after the first 20 years of the study and showed that lung volume, the vital capacity (VC), was the best parameter apart from age to predict when a subject would become ill or die. The vital capacity steadily declines with age, and the relationship between vital capacity and mortality is inversely related – the smaller the vital capacity, the shorter amount of time you have to live.

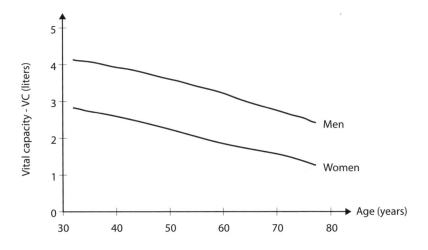

The vital capacity of the lungs continues to decline with age.

To talk about the association between illnesses and breathing is very much like discussing whether the chicken came before the egg. Have you gotten ill because you breathe incorrectly, or are you breathing incorrectly because you are ill? However, there is no doubt about the fact that breathing effectively will boost your body and your immune system and thus help you avoid a number of illnesses and unpleasant symptoms.

In healthy persons, illnesses are often caused by weakened or stiff muscles within the breathing mechanism. The same phenomenon can be observed in individuals that have broken their arm and have it in a cast for four to six weeks. The muscles of the arm will have become smaller and weaker and the joints of the arm will become very stiff. Similarly, if the muscles of your upper body are not kept active, the breathing capacity of the lungs will be significantly reduced. In the same way a weak nervous system will prevent efficient breathing, particularly if the central breathing regulator in the brain has been incorrectly programmed after several years of "abuse". Whether incorrect breathing or a reduced lung function causes serious illness, the consequence is that many secondary illnesses will follow.

Health perception

There is a great historical and cultural difference between modern and traditional health treatments. Despite the rapid technological development, modern medical treatment is often stuck in dualistic thinking, in which the mind is separated from the body – a way of thinking that can be traced through history to great thinkers such as Locke and Descartes and even further back to Aristotle and Plato in ancient Greece. However, in the latter half of the 1800's philosophers and physicians questioned dualism; and from the American psychologist, William James, theories about the psyche were published in 1890, where the human mind finally met the brain and the rest of the body.

In spite of these thoughts, traditional Western medicine continues to be reactive, not proactive. In other words it treats symptoms, but not the causes. Subsequently, diagnoses are often considered as distinct physical phenomena and treated accordingly. Contrary to medical traditions of Western culture, the philosophy and view of man in Asia is often more holistic. This is evident for instance in the Indian science of *Ayurveda* that assigns a crucial role to the interaction between a healthy diet and an active lifestyle. The same applies to yoga where the focus is on the breath.

"It is better to prevent than cure"

In Chinese culture a similar holistic view of health and illness exists, where body and mind are connected e.g. in meditation and acupuncture. I have been told that doctors in ancient China were not paid in accordance with the number of patients they treated, but the number of patients they kept healthy. Perhaps this would be an interesting approach to adopt in our society!

The more details of the body and mind functions that modern science describes, the more fascinated I become with regards to the wealth of knowledge that lies hidden in ancient Asian wisdom. Understanding the link between body, mind, soul and the surrounding universe is impressive, and I recommend everybody, professionals as well as laymen, to read the ancient Indian scriptures.

Here I draw a sharp line between Modern science and traditional Asian traditions. However, let me point out that I do not consider modern Western health sciences solely as mechanical and rigid, just as I do not see pink lotus flowers before my inner eye every time I think about Asian traditions. But when the best of two worlds fuse in symbiosis, I do believe that we can only benefit from the outcome.

Fortunately, I sense a new and greater openness to the health aspects of non-Western cultures, and a number of biological and medical studies have validated the Asian holistic approach in recent years. One good example is acupuncture, which was regarded as pure voodoo just 20 years ago by Western physicians, but today it is accepted and applied to a wide range of treatments performed by doctors, dentists and physiotherapists. Relaxation techniques such as mindfulness and other forms of meditation flood us like a true wellness-wave, which is possibly both fortunate and desired. On this same wave arises activities such as pilates and yoga, though unfortunately with a backlog of the 80s and 90s, which focused on fitness and bodybuilding.

However, regardless of the many new achievements and positive trends, a focus on that which binds the body, brain and heart together - the breath - is still missing, but it is dawning on us as we are becoming better at listening to our environment and to nature's breath. Ancient methods, such as *tai chi* and *qi gong*, are gaining ground in modern society. We need to become better at listening to ourselves and to fill our lungs with vitalizing oxygen and energy-rich prana. The more air we inhale, the more energy and life we gain. An appropriate point to mention is that *chi* and *qi* are synonymous with the word prana, the energy of everything.

A healthy and efficient breathing will keep us fit and make us recover faster from illnesses. Breathing is free and can be used in any context. Breathing techniques are employed in maternity hospitals, but it is not only during birth that efficient breathing is essential - it is also essential to maintain life. As far as I know, breathing techniques are employed only peripherally in modern health care, for example by individual physiotherapists and at special epilepsy clinics, but they have enormous therapeutic potential in many fields.

If doctors, nurses, physiotherapists and other health workers had a better understanding of the many possibilities that properly performed breathing exercises offer, they would be able to customize programs for patients that accurately match their illness and needs. This obviously requires time and effort, but I believe it would be common sense and economically viable in the long run.

Prevent illnesses

It is important for me to stress that I do not consider breathing a magical cure that with a touch of a wand will remove all sorts of illnesses or cure any serious disease. However, I do believe that an effective breath can heal, soothe, and even prevent illnesses in many situations.

> "By proper practice of pranayama all diseases are eradicated. Through improper practice all diseases can arise."
>
> HATHA YOGA PRADIPIKA

Many are familiar with the adverse consequences of a poor breathing technique, while very few are aware of the benefits of efficient breathing. This is especially unfortunate since breathing exercises can help healthy people remain healthy and help sick people to become healthy faster. When you are ill and weakened, you are usually less active or simply passive. Particularly in connection with more serious diseases, patients are often bedridden and thus do not move at all, which can lead to further bodily decline.

The human body is not adapted to lying motionless, and clear signs of deterioration are evident after a few days of inactivity. The heart loses its strength, muscles become weak and even the skin begins to deteriorate. The lungs also lose their elasticity especially for diseases that involve fluid retention (edema) or degradation of the alveoli such as smoker's lungs or pneumonia.

The breath is an ideal tool for debilitated or bedridden patients, since it offers boundless possibilities to counteract the degeneration of the body. And the amazing part is that the breath is always at hand. With simple breathing exercises anyone can perform circuit-, flexibility- and cardio-training. By this I mean that most of the muscles in your upper body will be activated and stretched. The same applies to the diaphragm, which is the central pumping muscle responsible for efficient breathing.

When you practice breathing, the lungs are strengthened while the chest is made more elastic, and thus breathing becomes more effective. This means that it becomes more economical and minimizes the amount of oxygen required for breathing. The oxygen saved can then be used elsewhere in the body where there is more need for it, such as to combat inflammation and other conditions. Concurrently, training your breath will improve your fitness, because elevating your breathing frequency will raise the pulse, increase blood flow in the body and thus exercise and strengthen your heart. And all this can be achieved without moving an inch. It will also stimulate all the internal organs and digestion, and thus cleanse, create balance and vitalize.

The only breathing exercise that I know of being practiced in Danish hospitals is the so-called PEEP flow. This method is primarily employed for patients with pulmonary diseases. The patient blows air through a small tube thereby increasing air resistance. This will lead to an increased internal lung pressure and thus oxygen tension; in addition, it helps to strengthen the respiratory muscles. In effect, the small air-filled alveoli expand and more oxygen can be absorbed into the bloodstream.

A CPAP mask (CPAP stands for Continuous Positive Airway Pressure) has the same effect. It provides a small positive pressure in the airways. The same technique as PEEP and CPAP is exploited by freedivers, when they prepare for a dive. The technique is called "purge-breathing" and air resistance is created using the tongue, by closing the lips or by placing a finger on the mouth upon exhalation. This is just an example of how breath training can be simplified without compromising effect. The technique avoids the use of a device and is more practical and accessible during hospitalization as well as outside of the hospital.

The activation of the entire nervous system is also important, and the breath's incredible and immediate effect on the mental state is perhaps the most important factor. Furthermore, breathing exercises can provide a meaningful activity for bedridden patients that can be performed anytime and break the monotony of hospitalization.

It would be beneficial to give a general explanation of how and why various breathing techniques can be beneficial during a course of treatment. It is also relevant to look more closely at how the body reacts physically and mentally to different breathing exercises.

Use your nose!

I have repeatedly emphasized the importance of breathing through your nose. This applies to everybody, everywhere and at any time. There are numerous reasons for this, but here follows a physiological and very tangible explanation.

A couple of years ago in Sweden a simple but ingenious experiment was conducted. It was discovered that blood is oxygenated 10-15% more, when you breathe through the nose compared to breathing through your mouth. The explanation was due to the release of nitrogen oxide (NO) from the sinuses that are in contact with the nasal cavity through small openings.

When you breathe through your nose, NO flows with the inhaled air into the lungs where it makes the blood vessels in the alveoli expand. This allows a greater volume of blood to pass, whereby more oxygen can be taken up. When NO was given to those who breathed through the mouth, the same effect was registered. This showed that it is actually NO which mediates the marked rise in oxygenation.

It is problematic when people breathing through a respirator have a tube fitted directly to their trachea, because the nose is bypassed. In the study a simple pump sucked air from one of the nostrils of the patient and mixed it with the air of the respirator, which increased oxygenation of the blood by 10-20%.

This study firmly establishes the importance of breathing through the nose, but it is also another beautiful example of how easily and cheaply a standard treatment can be modified and improved. Likewise, it illustrates that treatment with air or pure oxygen may not always be the best solution. Treatment-wise, it is not only patients using respirators that can benefit from NO's ability to widen blood vessels. It also applies to patients suffering serious chronic illnesses such as high blood pressure (hypertension), pulmonary complications, cardiovascular diseases or those who have suffered a stroke.

NO is also one of the active ingredients of nitroglycerine that is used as a heart medicine because it causes the blood vessels of the heart to relax and expand.

You may be familiar with the fact that heart patients, if feeling ill, can place a nitroglycerine pill under their tongue, because this compound rapidly enters the blood stream through the mucosa. I have no idea how long this procedure has existed in the West, but I know that it was described in Chinese medicine about 1,000 years ago. The recipe was discovered in a Buddhist cave at Dunhuang, and some of the scripture reads: "Putting under the tongue, to cause heart qi to flow freely. For treating symptoms such as struck by evil, acute heart pains and cold in the hands and feet which can kill a patient in an instant. (...) This is a sure cure." Note that the scriptures use the term qi, which as we noted earlier is identical with the Indian concept of prana – life energy, the power of the universe. Here the expression is used in a very specific context, and it makes sense since qi is precisely the energy that allows a terminally ill patient to regain vitality. This is a perfect example of East meeting West in the true spirit of yoga – even if it took 1,000 years to build this bridge!

In addition, it should also be mentioned that NO has many other beneficial effects. It has a strong antibacterial effect, and can kill both bacteria and viruses. Indeed, studies have shown that NO successfully eliminates bacteria such as *Salmonella* and *Shigella* as well as other bacteria that often affect patients with pulmonary diseases caused by smoking or cystic fibrosis. Thus, the effect is not limited to an improved oxygenation of blood: the immune system is also spared and strengthened.

Furthermore, NO also has an amazing property, which reduces oxygen consumption of the cells without compromising the overall energy production. This quite peculiar quality is obviously beneficial to anyone, but particularly to people who are sick and need to optimize oxygen utilization in every conceivable way to become healthy quickly.

Pranayama prescribed

Today it is quite legitimate for doctors to prescribe physical exercise to their patients. This is a brilliant initiative, but it is also a typical modern way of thinking - that exercise can only do you good. But this is not necessarily the case, because if the recommended exercise is not of the right kind, and if the intended "dose" is inappropriate, exercise can do more harm than good, either by stressing the body physically or simply by being yet another "thing" that has to be done during a busy and hectic day.

Exercise is not always the appropriate recipe to control weight. Overweight and obesity is to a great extent caused by personal problems, social heritage and bad habits rather than bad genes, although many people often use the latter as an excuse. Frankly, I believe it would be extremely beneficial to consider these facts more soberly. Of course, exercise can be an excellent and motivational tool for weight loss, but I think it is a better strategy to say that you wish to lose weight to be able to exercise – not the other way round. This calls for a change of attitude regarding life, and this is what a healthy and sincere diet is really all about.

The focus of this book lies in a conscious and controlled breathing, which is precisely the core of the various techniques within the discipline of pranayama. It boils down to regulating the breath and thereby the energy of life, prana. Some of the pranayama exercises activate the calming nervous system and are beneficial against stress and fatigue, whereas other exercises stimulate the stress-activating nervous system and thus energize and enhance metabolism.

If the exercises are combined properly, you will be able to harmonize the two opposing parts of the autonomous nervous system, and thereby create a better balance in the body as well as the mind. Pranayama does not only influence the autonomous nervous system but also the part of the nervous system that is under the control of the will, as ob-

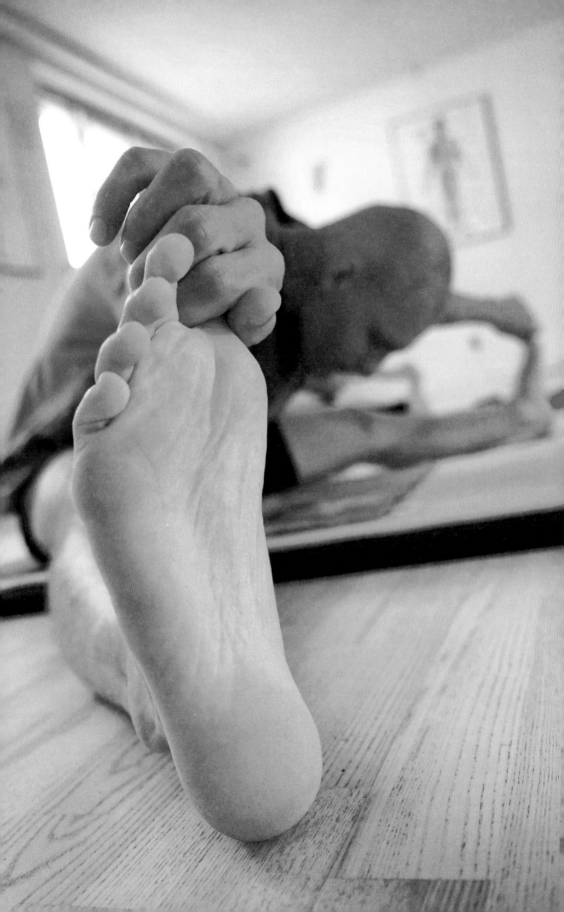

served in tests on the strength used in handshakes. This aspect makes pranayama an obvious tool for strengthening the nerve-muscle coupling, and is thus suitable in connection with rehabilitation programs, described in a case study at the end of this chapter. Unfortunately, pranayama techniques are not widely applied and hence not employed in health care treatments. I hope that pranayama will become integrated in health care practices in the future and be prescribed by physicians. Let us turn to the physiological mechanisms modern science has in recent years identified as being a part of pranayama's positive and powerful impact on our organism.

The primary mechanism of pranayama is to activate the lungs and thus the entire respiratory system, leading to a strengthened blood and lymph circulatory system. A deep, slow and controlled pranayama breath is believed to affect the body through receptors in the tissue of the lung that are activated when the lung wall is stretched beyond the normal breathing capacity. Furthermore, receptors in the muscles of the abdomen and diaphragm are believed to be involved in and affect the breathing rhythm, as do the smooth muscles in the lungs. The connective tissue surrounding the lungs is also influenced, and the overall effect is a shift in the autonomous nervous system leading to the calming parasympathetic part gaining control. The result is a lowered pulse, blood pressure and oxygen consumption. You are probably aware of the soothing and relaxing effect a long and deep sigh can have, when you have stretched your lungs and diaphragm.

Another beneficial effect of a slow and deep breath is the increased sensitivity of various receptors in the body that otherwise decline due to age, heart diseases or hypertension. Furthermore, this kind of breathing has a favorable impact on the body's hormone production, nervous system and immune response. Another important and well-documented effect of pranayama is a shift in brain oscillations, generating a greater degree of relaxation and well-being.

Pranayama's greatest force, however, lies in the regulatory effect of the exercises on the lung-heart-brain connection that not only becomes balanced but also synchronized. Pranayama is a very complex discipline, since it affects the body through the entire nervous system and exactly because of this omnipotence it is an obvious therapeutic tool that can be adapted to specific diseases and patient demands.

Pranayama has proven particularly effective in cases of illnesses related to mental disorders. In both children and adults with mental disabilities, breathing exercises have been shown to improve intelligence, learning ability, social behavior and the general psychological profile.

Increased awareness, enhanced mental focus, a sense of being calm and composed, and an improved stress tolerance are also positive effects of a relaxed and correct breath, which has been used successfully to treat people with lapses in concentration. Therefore, pranayama is an obvious candidate for the treatment of Attention Deficit Hyperactive Disorder (ADHD).

Recently it has been estimated that nearly 5% of American adults are affected by ADHD, and they usually are not aware that they suffer ADHD. Particularly, pranayama exercises that focus on long breath holds and slow exhalation combined with different forms of concentration and meditation are likely to be effective against this disorder. The powerful activation of the vagus nerve by pranayama exercises and the mental and physical calmness it mediates has made it a successful tool in the treatment of depressed patients and patients suffering psychosocial and post traumatic stress. This agrees with recent research that indicates that stress and depression are closely related. So it is not surprising that an activation of the calming part of the nervous system and an improved mental balance have a positive effect.

Some Danish epilepsy clinics have employed breathing exercises as a preventive treatment. This is an extremely positive trend, which will hopefully soon spread to the rest of the health care system.

As described, one of the main parameters of pranayama is the direct affect on the vagus nerve. This vagal activation of the calming part of the nervous system has been known and used in yoga for several thousand years, but has only caught the attention of Western physicians within the last decade. Still, better late than never. Let us take a closer look at how the vagus nerve may serve therapeutic purposes.

The importance of the vagus nerve

For almost a century neurologists have been aware of the fact that some seizures and heart disorders can be stopped by applying pressure to the carotid artery. The pressure activates the vagus nerve which arises in the brain stem, where the breathing and heart rhythm are regulated. It sends off nerve branches to the throat, lungs, heart and many other visceral organs of the body. Recent studies performed on animals have shown that stimulating the vagus nerve electrically can reduce epileptic seizures, and since 1997 vagus nerve stimulation (VNS) has been used on humans.

The method is relatively simple and consists of a small device that is implanted in the chest. A wire extends from the device to the throat where it is in direct contact with the vagus nerve. Approximately every five minutes a low voltage current is conducted to the nerve which then sends a message to the area in the brain that controls the respiratory rhythm, sleep, mood and seizures. The patient can even activate the device if an epileptic seizure is on the way.

Stimulating the vagus nerve has also proved to be an effective deterrent against the eating disorder *bulimia* (overeating followed by vomiting), and thus a good alternative to medical treatment. In addition, vagal stimulation also appears to have a beneficial effect in women who suffer from nausea during pregnancy, whereby medications that may affect the fetus are avoided. The VNS implant is a small metal rod that is implanted in the neck near the vagus nerve. The metal rod can be controlled from the outside and works on the same principle as described for epilepsy.

Stimulating the vagus nerve electrically with a weak current is, at any rate, a more gentle approach than using drugs, but a natural stimulation and regulation of the vagus nerve should be preferred. The most useful, safe and accessible methods are obviously the thousand-year old breathing exercises.

When performing prolonged dives in freediving it is possible to experience a "samba" which is reminiscent of an epileptic seizure. A samba can occur when the oxygen level in your body is low. By using special breathing techniques and combining them with an intake of different elements that affect the nervous system, such incidents can be prevented or mitigated, even when oxygen levels are low. This phenomenon could be worth examining closer.

Vibration therapy for body and mind

One may argue that all stimuli received by the vagus nerve and the visceral organs occur as a result of vibrations. Everything vibrates, even this seemingly solid book you have in your hands is one big atomic dance party! "Healing" music is already being employed in many hospitals, and this kind of therapy aims directly at lowering heart rate and creating calming brain waves.

The magic of sounds is that they consist of waves that can be more or less harmonized. If sounds oscillate uniformly, they create vibrations and develop a "resonance" in various parts of the body. Sound is waves of energy and this energy is like a stimulating and vitalizing micro-massage to your cells. When all the cells in your body vibrate in their optimal frequency, they work most effectively. The goal of yoga is to expand your consciousness to such an extent that it fuses and becomes one with the Universe – the state called samadhi or nirvana. It happens exactly when the vibrations and energy of your cells synchronize with the rhythm of nature, which is controlled by prana – the universal energy of life.

More and more research is focusing on examination of the many complex mechanisms that music contains and the beneficial impact that different sounds have on our brain, and in turn our state of mind. This is a positive indication of openness and desired innovations are beginning to see the light of day. However, an easy method exists, which is effortless to practice and entirely without risk - simply using the waves of sound produced by your own vocal chords. Different sounds depending on where and what they are to affect can be used. Close your eyes for a moment and say the sacred mantra Om (or Aum) out loud and clear three times – and hold the tone as long as possible. Om is pronounced "AAUUMMMMM" and it creates vitalizing vibrations throughout your body – especially in your lungs, heart, neck, jaw, tongue and brain. You may also generate a long and soft Amen which produces similar oscillations and has an immediate soothing effect.

In yoga, great significance is ascribed to being able to stimulate the calming part of the nervous system by means of sounds, since it is an effective way to create a link between body, mind, emotions, intellect and the energy flow of prana. It vitalizes, transforms and heals each and every cell in our body simultaneously.

Another example of useful sounds that are particularly beneficial to the body is a clean "A" or "O" sound which will make the chest, sternum and neck vibrate. Vibrations in the sternum will stimulate the immune system because the oscillations boost the *thymus*, a small gland in the chest which controls the production of the body's key defence cells called *T lymphocytes*. The thymus becomes smaller and smaller with age and almost disappears in the end. Some researchers even believe that different infections and cancers in old people are closely linked to the decline in T lymphocyte production. Hence, if you were to stimulate the thymus in some way e.g. through prayer or song, it is sure to be advantageous. Elderly people as well as ill people following a treatment need a strong immune system.

Vibrations in the throat will stimulate another important gland, the *thyroid*. This gland produces hormones that regulate metabolism and thus the body's energy consumption and body weight. In addition, it also assists in strengthening heart function. Apart from the fact that you can stimulate this gland to some extent with vibrations, a combination of generating sounds and using the yoga shoulder stand, can create additional stimulation. This is partly due to an increased blood flow to the neck and head, and secondly, because the natural *Throat Lock* that this posture creates increases the pressure in the thyroid, giving it a gentle massage.

Another outcome of vibrations in the throat and the resulting vagus nerve stimulation is the immediate reduction in blood pressure and number of heartbeats. People with heart conditions or patients who have suffered a heart attack can combine breathing exercises with sound generation as a simple preventive or therapeutic method.

I have spoken to Italian physicians about initiating a new project where breathing exercises are included in the treatment of stroke. Cardiologist Alessandro Pingitore from the National Research Council (CNR) in Pisa has already developed a method that he believes would be worth testing in Denmark and Italy. We have discussed a number of possible solutions for a better, safer and cheaper treatment for these cardiac patients. Furthermore, he sent me an interesting note in which he reflects on heart treatment. I sincerely hope that the future status of the planet's throbbing hearts is brighter than forecasts predict. At present, cardiac and cardiovascular diseases are the main causes of death worldwide.

"Cardiovascular therapy is primarily aimed at the heart. In the case of acute myocardial infarction, the large blood vessels are opened, and operation is conducted if the heart valves function incorrectly.

However, it is important to remember that the heart is part of the complex and highly organized system that comprises the human organism. This means that a malfunction in the heart affects the whole system. As proof of this, we can observe that people with heart attacks are more likely to have depression, just as people with depression are more likely to have heart attacks.

A holistic approach combined with a conventional treatment may therefore be advantageous to patients with heart diseases. In this respect, relaxation and breathing exercises are particularly obvious choices, because they affect the entire human organism through the central nervous system, endocrine system and immune system.

In this respect, the experience of athletes like Stig Åvall Severinsen is valuable, since relaxation and breathing exercises are used to achieve a greater understanding of oneself. In other words, the awareness of capacity and limitations are increased which improves the extreme sports performance. When we regard an illness as an extreme experience, or even better as an experience that lies beyond the normal life, we will also understand the potential benefits that relaxation and breathing exercises from the holistic approach can offer, in addition to the conventional "state of the art" treatment."

Alessandro Pingitore
Institute of Clinical Physiology, Pisa

Another interesting significance of breathing while using your voice is simply that the breathing frequency is lowered and the natural breath becomes longer. The same happens when you hum or sing, which as you know, causes a feeling of happiness and well-being.

Asthma *can* be cured by training

Many people are struck with asthma during their life, but how do you live with asthma without it taking up your whole life?

A genuine arsenal of hormone-containing inhalers and pills that can alleviate an asthma attack already exists. Unfortunately, these medications do not cure asthma. Although they are good at relieving the symptoms, they can lead to secondary adverse effects that sometimes force patients to take more and more medication because of the body's reaction.

Over a dinner at a research conference in Pisa in the spring of 2008 I sat next to a female doctor who treated patients with asthma. She explained that the asthma patients used a variety of hormone products according to individual needs. I asked her if they used breathing techniques such as pranayama or *Buteyko* at her clinic, but this was not the case. She acknowledged that she had never heard that breathing exercises could have a beneficial effect on asthma.

Frankly, I was somewhat surprised because I knew of several examples of freedivers in my club in Aarhus who had cut down significantly on their use of medication. This was mainly due to the fact that as freedivers they constantly trained new breathing techniques – both slow and controlled breathing and prolonged breath holds. Moreover, I came to know of several cases where people were able to leave all of their medications on the shelf, including Peter Wurschy, a Dutch freediver and champion in distance diving who suffered severe chronic asthma for years, but today is completely free of symptoms.

"I got asthma after a prolonged infection that I contracted during a trip through India. In the beginning it was not too bad, but after some months, breathing became increasingly difficult when I went for a run or the environment was cold or dusty.

I went to a doctor and after I had my lungs X-rayed and a lung function test, I received my first medicine, which was *salbutamol*, an inhalant. In the beginning I only used it once a day, but after a while it was sometimes necessary to use it three-five times daily. I went to the doctor again: this time he prescribed a new medication (*salmeterol*), also to inhale. I used it twice daily and salbutamol when necessary.

I was a scuba diver at the time. However, the doctor forbade me this after a new lung examination. Asthma and scuba diving was a "no go". I was looking for a new sport and took up freediving and started training my lungs with yoga breaths and pranayama. After six months it was no longer necessary to use salbutamol, but I still had to take my other medication. However, I used it less and less and usually only in the morning.

I continued my annual visits to the doctor, and after a long test the doctor said that my lungs were getting stronger and produced less mucus. I asked whether I could start scuba diving again, which he still forbade me.

The following year my test results were even better, and I was finally allowed to take up scuba diving again. However, I had to inhale my salbutamol before I jumped into the water.

After the third year, my asthmatic symptoms had disappeared. My doctor asked me to perform the lung function test three times, and he could see that my lungs were normal again. He even sent me back to the hospital to take a major test, since he could not believe that such a change was possible.

I particularly train breath holds and perform long dives."

Peter Wurschy, 38
Instructor at the Apnea Academy, Amsterdam

Naturally, the many hormone-based products have their justification, and there is no doubt that they help millions of people to have a better everyday life. Nonetheless, it is still unfortunate that there is so little emphasis on natural cures.

A number of scientific studies have shown that yoga and pranayama in particular have a positive effect on patients suffering from asthma. Even breathing exercises in their simple form with a 1:2 ratio i.e. an exhalation that is twice as long as the inhalation, have been shown to produce a beneficial effect. In some studies, progress can be observed within a week, although a treatment program for asthma is often long-term and depends on whether the asthma patient continues with the exercises in their everyday life. In the best cases, asthma symptoms completely vanish, and in many cases medication can be reduced, fitness rating is increased and lung performance is improved.

Optimized breathing

As a child I suffered a kind of asthma, which was probably triggered by my beloved guinea pigs. Luckily, I grew out of this asthma, but in some instances breathing can become strenuous e.g. if I train hard in chlorinated water or when running in winter.

Once when my younger brother took me on a mountain bike ride in the forest and tempted me up a very steep hill, I experienced an asthma attack. Since the weather was cold and I gave myself fully to the challenge, my breathing became a wheezing when I got to the top of the hill. Quite spontaneously, I took a few deep hook breaths which gave an immediate soothing effect. Hook breathing is simply to fill your lungs completely and hold the inhalation by shutting the air off in the throat while pushing air upward using the diaphragm and abdominal muscles. This increases air pressure in the lungs and dilates the airways – bronchial tubes, bronchiole and the small alveoli. Try the technique yourself, if you experience a similar asthma attack.

I am by no means an expert on asthma, but just want to outline why it actually makes sense that breathing exercises, especially slow exhalation and simple breath holding pauses, can relieve and sometimes cure asthma. If you try to breathe slowly and with control you can achieve a higher concentration of carbon dioxide in the lungs as well as in the blood vessels. Since carbon dioxide expands blood vessels in the lungs and the rest of the body, it has a beneficial effect. It also seems very likely that carbon dioxide can help to recalibrate the control center of the breathing rhythm in the brain stem. In other words, re-establish a healthy and natural breathing frequency and depth.

The gas molecule nitrogen oxide (NO) that we know is activated through the nose also contributes to relaxation and to expand blood vessels, like carbon dioxide. Add to this an antibacterial function, which can help to improve local conditions in an irritated lung. To further increase the concentration of NO – and thus the dilation of blood vessels – humming sounds during nose breathing can advantageously be employed. This rather special kind of breathing is beneficial because the buzzing sound has been shown to increase the concentration of NO in the nasal cavity up to 15 times, since the air in the nose more readily mixes with NO-rich air from the sinuses.

Moreover, the simple pressure equalizing *Valsalva maneuver* can help as it presses air from the lungs to all the cavities in the skull, and there are indeed a lot around the nose and forehead. During a strong cold or if you have swum under water with a blocked nose, you may have experience a marked pain in the sinuses. The Valsalva maneuver is easy to perform and everyone can perform it right away, because it requires no prior knowledge. Close your mouth, pinch your nose shut and push air up in your head using your diaphragm and abdominal muscles. You may be able to hear air whistling through the *eustachian tubes* to the eardrum (psssttt).

The technique is widely used in diving, flying, mountain driving or in any instance where you need to equalize the pressure in your ears. If you maintain the air from the lungs in your head for 20-30 seconds after the Valsalva maneuver, a substantial amount of NO is added to the air, which can then be drawn into the lungs.

Another exercise that will also be beneficial to asthmatics is the alternate nostril breathing. In this exercise inhalation and exhalation constantly alternate from one nostril to the other, which cleans the entire nose and enhances NO absorption. It would be particularly effective to make the pause between the inhalation and exhalation longer than usual and even close both nostrils with the fingers simultaneously, as this will elevate the concentration of carbon dioxide as well as NO and contribute to the benefits described above.

Oxygen treatment

There is no doubt that oxygen is vital to every cell in the body. It is a well-known fact in the sports world that the body can achieve better results with more oxygen in the blood. But how do you get the natural oxygen content in the body to increase permanently? There is reason to believe that it can be done through treatments with oxygen under pressure.

In a study involving a group of Italian freedivers in 1999, the Belgian doctor in neurophysiology, Constantino Balestra, discovered that the divers' content of the oxygen binding molecule hemoglobin in the red blood cells had increased by 14% after five days of training with three daily dives to 40 meters of depth. At this depth the pressure is five times higher than at the surface, and oxygen tension in the lungs of the freedivers increased fivefold. Since the atmospheric air in the freedivers' lungs contains 20% oxygen, a person standing on land would have to breathe 100% pure oxygen to create the same conditions in the body.

The elevated blood values that Doctor Balestra observed, lead him to investigate whether there was a closer correlation between oxygen tension and the increased production of red blood cells. An obvious "candidate" to explain the increase was the natural hormone EPO, which exists in the body and stimulates the formation of new red blood cells.

Doctor Balestra then had 16 healthy subjects breathe 100% oxygen for a period of two hours under normal pressure conditions. To his great surprise he was able to measure a 60% increase in EPO concentration in the blood after 36 hours. So the investigation suggested that inspiring pure oxygen at normal pressure conditions stimulated the production of EPO.

Treating patients with oxygen at a level higher than atmospheric pressure (hyperbaric oxygen therapy) is also gaining more ground. In the pressure chamber at the Copenhagen University Hospital oxygen pressure treatment is used for wound healing and various forms of inflammation.

In one promising story in particular, I met a small boy named Frederik who was treated with oxygen. When Frederik was one and a half years old he was diagnosed with cerebral palsy, which is an umbrella term comprising a variety of physical disabilities where the brain's ability to control the muscles does not function properly. Generally physicians were very reluctant to lay down any prediction or even a helping hint. The very pessimistic senior physician, who had Frederik's case, thought it would be an achievement if he were to sit without assistance some day.

Frederik's mother then had Frederik treated with acupuncture, and Frederik slowly began to develop skills. In the summer of 2006 his parents read about a special kind of oxygen treatment, Hyperbaric Oxygen Therapy (HBOT), which is roughly the same treatment that divers suffering decompression sickness receive. In Britain this kind of treatment has been used to treat multiple sclerosis (a nerve disease that affects the brain and spinal cord) for more than 25 years and has within recent years also been conducted on children with cerebral palsy. Frederik's parents contacted Professor Philip James of Dundee in Scotland, who is a specialist within this field, to inquire whether it was possible to treat

Frederik in Scotland. In January 2007 they went to stay in Dundee for a month to have Frederik treated with HBOT.

Before they left, Frederik could walk only with splints on both legs and with the help of a walker for balance. After just three weeks in Scotland, he could walk without his walker. He experienced many bonus effects from the treatment and his energy level was also boosted. As a result, his parents decided to spend yet another month in Dundee in the summer of 2007. Again there were notable results from the treatment. Frederik could suddenly walk without his splints and continues to do so, though with orthopedic shoes to support his development. Subsequently, his parents have invested in their own portable oxygen chamber, which continually benefits Frederik.

Can oxygen relieve cancer?

Oxygen treatment, both with and without pressure, has yielded some promising results in recent years, particularly in cancer treatment. One example of this is of a female patient with stage III breast cancer who received 100% oxygen a few times a day during her chemotherapy treatment. Chemotherapy treatment had made the hemoglobin level in her blood drop, but the oxygen treatment quickly raised it again.

The same effect could have been achieved by injecting quantities of the hormone EPO, which stimulates the formation of red blood cells. Apart from being very expensive this procedure can sometimes lead to an unfortunate immune response. Increasing EPO levels through the body's own natural mechanisms by subjecting the patient to 100% oxygen is simple, safe, inexpensive and an easy method that can be readily implemented in dealing with a range of cancers.

A Norwegian study has recently shown that tumors in rats with breast cancer decreased 60% in size after a few treatments of 100% oxygen at normal and slightly elevated barometric pressure. Compare this with a roughly 36% decrease in tumor size in rats treated with a chemotherapy agent – only half as effective. Apart from the decrease in tumor size, a large increase in the number of dead cancer cells was measured after the pure oxygen treatment.

It is interesting that something as simple as breathing pure oxygen can be used effectively against something as serious and draining to the body as cancer. If pushed to extremes, these studies indicate that if you were stranded on a deserted island and had cancer, the best thing you could do for yourself would be to perform breath holds and dive as much as possible preferably to about 40 or 50 meters.

It must be noted that oxygen treatment is far from being a new "invention". Already in the 1920s the Nobel laureate Otto Warburg was a major proponent for the usefulness of copious amounts of oxygen in the fight against cancer. Otto Warburg was interested in the energy processes of the individual cell's "breathing" (respiration), and he believed that normal cells were transformed into cancer cells when they were fed less oxygen than normal. In lectures he said: "Cancer, above all other diseases, has countless secondary causes. But, even for cancer, there is only one prime cause. Summarized in a few words, the prime cause of cancer is the replacement of the respiration of oxygen in normal body cells by the fermentation of sugar."

Another great supporter of the many applications of oxygen therapy was the German physicist, Manfred von Ardenne. He developed an impressively systematic and thorough approach to cancer treatment and gave several specific examples of oxygen treatment on lung cancer as well as bone cancer. One of his main theses was that low oxygen tensions in the body causes the normal micro-circulation of blood, oxygen and nutrients to change in some cells, which then may develop into cancer cells. The problem will be particularly pertinent near the venous blood vessels that carry oxygen-poor blood from the body back to the heart. Therefore he recommended cancer patients to take large quantities of antioxidants and to stimulate the production of red blood cells in addition to oxygen treatment, all of which contribute to a better oxidation of the body.

More oxygen with pranayama

Some simple pranayama exercises are ideal for oxygen treatment. Especially the exercises that have an element of hyperventilation and thus lower the concentration of carbon dioxide in the blood stream (e.g. the two exercises *Bellows Breathing* and *Brain Purification*).

The oxygen-depleted blood in the venous system, which runs to the heart, is significantly oxygenated by hyperventilation, and since 80% of the body's blood is in the venous system this may have a positive effect on the cells.

In contrast, hyperventilation does not have a major impact on the blood in the arterial system, which flows from the heart and carries oxygen to the cells, as it is already near saturation. This field has, to my knowledge, not received much attention, but it does pose some interesting possibilities. Some physicians may believe that exercises or studies like these are inappropriate, but in the fight against cancer I believe that all possibilities should be sought.

It seems reasonable that high oxygen concentrations can be an effective means to increase the energy system of the cells. A greater volume of atmospheric air can also be useful, if you know how!

Lung packing – a simple method to a better life

In recent years I have held a number of lectures for people who suffer injuries to the spinal cord or who have cerebral palsy. Common to many of these people is that they are confined to a wheelchair and therefore cannot move very much. Their lung function is often impaired which leaves them susceptible to lung complications and other secondary diseases. Besides talking about freediving, diving physiology and goal-setting during my lectures, I am also eager to teach these people some practical exercises that can stimulate or even increase their lung volume. As we have seen earlier, a larger lung volume is associated with a greater daily vitality and higher energy level, and not the least an opportunity to extend your life.

People who have suffered a fracture in the upper part of the neck or who suffer muscular dystrophy are restricted in the use of particularly their respiratory muscles. Therefore, the technique of lung packing, which can be used without activating the chest, is useful for this group of people. Even though this technique was described back in the early 1950s, knowledge of it is limited. Unfortunately, it is rarely used by the health care system in modern society, neither in connection with treatments, training or rehabilitation. This is a shame, and the reason why I am including the technique in this book.

"Lung packing" or "buccal pumping" is simple and anybody can learn it, though competent guidance is required. The key element of this maneuver is that it is the tongue, soft palate and larynx (vocal cords) that are used for breathing. Freedivers also employ this technique to pump more air into the lungs.

The first time I saw it was when I attended the Freediving World Cup in Nice in 2000. The French and the Spaniards call the technique "carpa", and it is probably the most suitable name because you really look like a carp gulping air.

This technique can be learned by anybody, if they receive proper instruction. Some people that suffer paralysis are self-taught – they learn the technique spontaneously. As with yoga, the body often

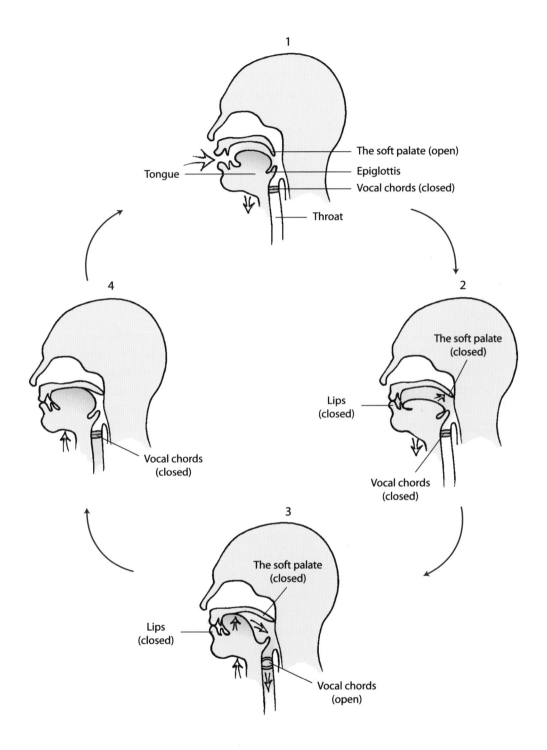

1

Tongue

The soft palate (open)

Epiglottis

Vocal chords (closed)

Throat

2

The soft palate (closed)

Lips (closed)

Vocal chords (closed)

3

The soft palate (closed)

Lips (closed)

Vocal chords (open)

4

Vocal chords (closed)

Applying the lung packing technique can fill the lungs with air without using the chest or diaphragm. Here the four phases are shown.

knows what to do if it is allowed. Indeed, some children use this technique when they dive (without prior knowledge of the technique), because they feel it helps them dive longer. They are right, and the technique is employed by all the reigning World Champion freedivers.

The principle is quite simple but requires proper coordination. The tongue is used as a piston to create a negative pressure, whereby a small amount of air is sucked into the mouth (like when you suck a straw), while the epiglottis is kept closed. The mouth is closed and the lips are held tightly together, whereupon you open to the trachea, while you push air into the lungs using the back of your tongue and sometimes the muscles in your cheeks. Then the lungs are shut off by sealing the throat, a new mouthful of air can be sucked in and the maneuver is repeated. You should not pack too many times, no more than 10 - 20 in a row – and even then only under competent supervision.

Lung packing has several advantages. The technique can relieve people who use mechanical ventilation for long periods (minutes, hours, all day) – they can talk louder, for a longer time, cry for help, cough phlegm up etc. It also makes it easier for them to engage in various activities and to lie down (without a ventilator), which facilitates care, therapy and training. Combined, these reliefs are motivational when learning lung packing. The method can also be used to expand the chest and stretch both chest and lung tissue, which increases the natural vital capacity of the lung. Along with increased energy and health, the technique also provides a higher degree of freedom.

A good friend and freediving colleague, Bill Strömberg, works as a breathing instructor for debilitated patients. When Bill instructs the patients, he divides the lung packing exercise up into small exercises that can be taught little by little. It is essential to achieve good control over the tongue, soft palate, epiglottis, vocal chords, throat etc. Once complete, coordination and strength are gained and the technique may be performed without problems. If the patients use a ventilator, they can leave it for a minute in the beginning, then two minutes and so on.

Bill told me about his first patient who was a boy with muscular dystrophy. His first spirometer test revealed a lung capacity of 300 ml, which is very little. After five lessons his capacity had risen to a liter, and after ten sessions it had increased to more than two liters representing a sevenfold increase. Imagine how much this boy can gain from life with such an increase in lung capacity.

Lung packing is a unique and simple method which is inexpensive to implement in different courses of treatments. Since, for obvious reasons, it can contribute to a whole new life with more independence and hence freedom, I hope it will spread.

Breath holding - tomorrow's "medicine"?

To hold your breath for a short period of time is simple and quite harmless if it is performed under the correct conditions. It is a very useful method, which positively influences a wide range of natural processes in the organism. Where suitable, holding the breath can be introduced to enhance existing courses of treatment.

Despite what many believe, breath holding is a natural part of breathing. It is simply the short break between inhalation and exhalation that can be prolonged by training, and which can benefit the entire body immensely.

Breath holding is more beneficial than most people immediately recognize. There still exists a widespread belief that breath holding is dangerous as well as harmful, but I hope you have a different opinion now that your knowledge about it has grown. A short breath hold in no way results in brain damage, because while you hold your breath plenty of oxygen circulates in your body, even though the concentration slowly declines during the breath hold.

In my body there is still more than 90% oxygen in my blood during the first five minutes. After six minutes oxygen concentration falls to about 80% and drops below the critical 50% only after eight or nine minutes. In other words, there is plenty of oxygen in the body in the several minutes after you initiate a breath hold. Damage to the brain only occurs at the moment when the brain has received too little oxygen for more than four minutes, either because the concentration of oxygen is too low i.e. below 50%, or because the blood flow in the brain has ceased e.g. in connection with a blood clot or heart attack. The brain does not die until it has been exposed to ten minutes without oxygen.

Even though you hold your breath for several minutes, there will be plenty of oxygen in the body and the heart will beat merrily. However, there are a number of other changes taking place in your body and many of them are actually extremely healthy, which several recent scientific studies document. You may even be tempted by the idea that it is natural to hold your breath now and then!

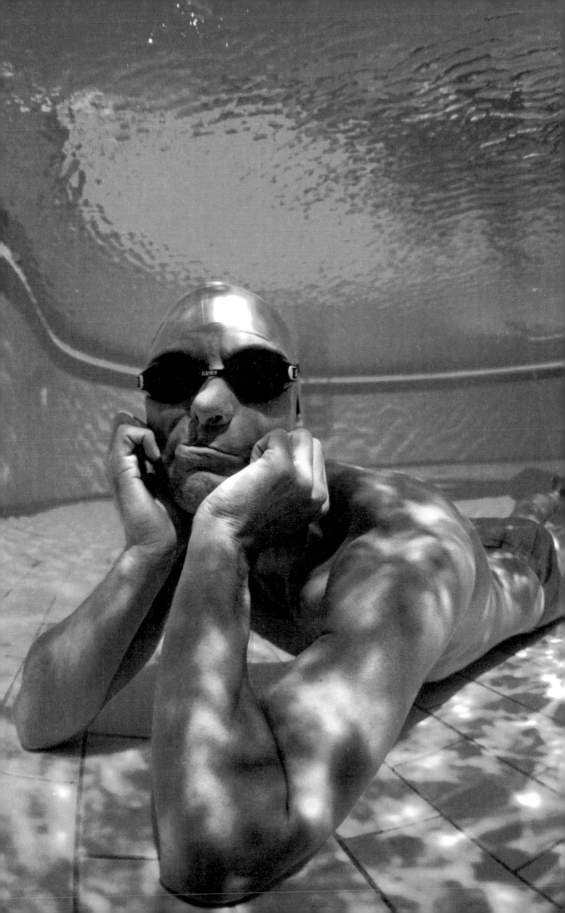

Breath holding can benefit and strengthen both brain, heart, lungs and blood.

A healthy response

When an organism is exposed to some sort of stress factor over a finite period, a lot of changes occur inside the many small factories of the cells that make the body more resilient to this specific stress factor in the future. This phenomenon is termed *preconditioning*, and you have observed it in your own body when you have been sunbathing. When summer begins you will quickly become red or burnt, because the cells of your skin have not been exposed to the sun during winter. After a few days with solar radiation your skin cells will pick up speed, form the protective substance *melatonin*, and be able to withstand more radiation without damage to the skin.

It depends on the stress factor as to which systems are upgraded inside the cells, but preconditioning is generally considered healthy. One stress factor has proven particularly good at making the cells alert, and this is variable concentrations of oxygen. It is not surprising that something as vital as oxygen deficiency can trigger a variety of modifications in the cell's interior, but their response is surprisingly great. If cells lack oxygen, the body immediately emits signals to utilize the available oxygen as good as possible: by activating the diving reflex, but also by directly changing the energy systems of each cell.

Experiments with rats and mice have shown that three hours of breathing air with 10% oxygen, as opposed to 21% in atmospheric air, protects the brain from serious damage that the experimental animals are subject to two days later. Hearts that are subject to a similar treatment demonstrate the same effect. In some cases the damage can be reduced by up to 30% in the preconditioned organ.

What is interesting in this context is that simple breath holding also creates a lower level of oxygen in the body. The same effect occurs when you travel to a higher altitude preferably above 2,000 meters, but it is not a very practical solution, especially for patients in a hospital. Prior to brain or heart surgery it would be advantageous to perform breath holds with different intervals. In this way the cells would be prepared for the stress of the surgery. Similarly, breath holding could be part of a rehabilitation program for people suffering a stroke of the brain or heart, because an optimization of the cell's ability to absorb oxygen during stress would be desirable.

It is also relevant to note that brief periods with low oxygen can have a long-term protective effect on the body's cells. Breath holding would also be a preventive agent in cases of chronic or acute low oxygen levels that often occur in the cardiovascular system of sick or elderly people.

Several recent studies have established that breath holding can increase the amount of red blood cells in the body. The immediate increase in the number of red blood cells is due to a contraction of the spleen, and the long-term increase, which is due to an increase in the concentration of the body's natural EPO concentration, increases the total pool of red blood cells. The significance of a greater quantity of red blood cells is not difficult to point out since they are responsible for delivering oxygen to the whole body.

Any illness will weaken the body to some extent, and the more oxygen carried to each individual cell, the faster the entire organism will recover. In diseases such as *anemia* (lack of red blood cells) or other conditions where the proportion of red blood cells are markedly weakened, breath holding would be particularly valuable. The uniqueness in this context is that the body produces a larger amount of EPO - preferable to the use of artificially produced EPO that can have unfortunate side effects.

With diseases that manifest themselves in the body, breath holding can be employed without risk. With mental disorders, notably depression, breath holding can undoubtedly also be used as a powerful and effective tool to create greater inner peace and joy, as it is in pranayama and meditation exercises. Although mental disorders are more complex to understand and deal with than physical illnesses, I believe that breath holding will come to play a role in future treatment of such diseases.

Self-help for diseases in the airways

We will now look at some of the diseases that can affect the airways and have a great impact on your general health. Different breathing techniques can actually cure some diseases, as we noted in connection with asthma. With regard to more serious illnesses such as advanced lung cancer, breathing exercises cannot cure in themselves. However, proper breathing will undoubtedly serve as an excellent preventive tool against any form of disease of the lungs and airways, relieve the course of the disease and provide energy and oxygen to the organism, if or when you become ill.

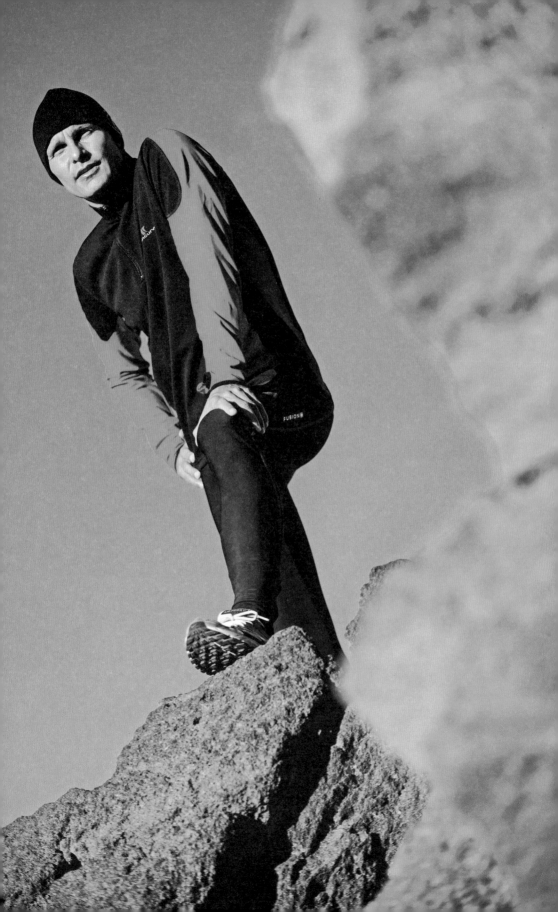

A slow and controlled breath will generally be beneficial for the following diseases. By particularly focusing on strength and flexibility in the diaphragm as well as the chest, the vital capacity of the lungs can be utilized optimally. As mentioned earlier, there is a direct correlation between the vital capacity (VC) and health, so the better the lungs are utilized, the better you will become – even during an illness.

Acute bronchitis

If an infection arises in the large bronchopulmonary branches, there will be an inflammation on the inside of the bronchi. This will lead to the formation of large amounts of mucus, which inhibit the free passage of air while increasing the risk that an infection will spread to the lungs.

Acute bronchitis will typically be accompanied by a shortness or a wheezing of the breath, slimy phlegm and chest pains, but the disease often disappears by itself after few days. In some cases, acute bronchitis can also worsen and develop into chronic bronchitis. Both forms of bronchitis fall within the category of "obstructive" lung diseases because they block a portion of the airways.

Breathing both more deeply and calmly will ventilate the lungs with more air. A special focus on the use of the diaphragm and a slow exhalation should be employed here, as these activate the vagus nerve and the soothing parasympathetic nervous system. Combined, this will lead to a relaxation and widening of the blood vessels and the muscles around the lungs, and thus ease the breathing.

Tuberculosis

Tuberculosis is the most common fatal infectious disease in the world today. It is caused by a mycobacterium that attacks the soft spongy alveolar tissue, and subsequently forms scars and holes called tubercles. *Tuberculin bacteria* actually exist in the lungs of many people who never develop tuberculosis. They can do so because a properly functioning immune system and proper breathing, which aerates the lungs thoroughly, will keep them down. It prevents the tuberculin bacteria from developing tuberculosis because they do not tolerate high oxygen concentrations. Today, tuberculosis is cured with antibiotics, as is the case with various forms of pneumonia.

Pneumonia

Pneumonia is often caused by *streptococcus* or *staphylococcus* bacteria. Symptoms of pneumonia are typically yellow or greenish phlegm that can be mixed with traces of blood. Typically, chest pains, coughing and fever are associated with the infection. Fluid will accumulate in the alveoli, which obviously reduces the respiratory surface that is exposed to air in the lungs resulting in shortness of breath and impaired breathing. In order to alleviate breathing, patients are often given a mask that supplies additional oxygen.

Smoker's lung (COPD)

In the US nearly 400,000 people die each year from tobacco-caused diseases, and COPD (*Chronic Obstructive Pulmonary Disease*) is the fourth leading cause of death. This is an alarmingly high figure. COPD is a term that covers a range of lung diseases, mostly caused by smoking and other particle pollutions. The symptoms are constant coughing, severe breathing difficulties and yellow or green phlegm.

A patient with COPD typically suffers chronic bronchitis and *emphysema* at the same time. Emphysema is a condition where the thin walls of the alveoli are degraded by chemical substances including tobacco smoke and other pollutants. When the air-filled alveoli are overstretched and burst due to decreased elasticity, the total respiratory surface is reduced. This inhibits both the uptake of oxygen and the excretion of carbon dioxide, which obviously is very serious for the body and can lead to cardiac arrest.

A calm, deep breath will often provide more oxygen and mental tranquillity for a patient, but naturally the best cure for smoker's lungs is to stop smoking – or at least to stop once the diagnosis is made.

Asthma

There has been a drastic increase in the number of patients with *asthma* in recent decades. Asthma affects almost 23 million Americans, including 7 million children according to the American Lung Association. Asthma rates in children under the age of five have increased more than 160% from 1980-1994 in America. Asthma may be inherited, but environmental factors may also play a key role. Asthma may be caused by food, pets, dust and obesity, but the exact cause is not known. Incorrect breathing may also lead to asthma. Many athletes also suffer from asthma, and this strongly suggests that breathing too much and/or too violently may irritate and abrade the airways and possibly alter the brain's breathing center, causing asthma.

Asthma is due to a hypersensitivity of the bronchi and bronchioles of the lungs, which swell and secrete extra mucus narrowing the air passage into the lungs. The disease can be treated with various hormone products, but unfortunately, these drugs cannot cure the disease. In some cases, pranayama breathing with slow exhalation, alternate nostril breathing and breath holding alleviate the symptoms or even cure asthma.

Sleep apnea

Short or long unconscious pauses in breathing during sleep is called *sleep apnea*. According to the National Institute of Health more than 12 million Americans are affected by sleep apnea. Sleep apnea and a disturbed sleep in general have a major affect on the whole body, particularly blood pressure and heart. Moreover, a restless sleep leads to fatigue, headaches and irritability during the day, and everything will seem more confusing, because the brain lacks sufficient rest and thus time to process and organize thoughts and sensory inputs from the previous day. In many cases sleep apnea is caused by obesity and is associated with severe snoring.

A conscious training of your breath in your everyday life will lead to a new regulation of the breathing rhythm that will become permanent and therefore follow the subconscious, when you sleep.

Lung cancer

Unfortunately, lung cancer is a very common form of cancer and the most deadly. By far, the majority of lung cancer is caused by smoking, which destroys the innermost cells in the bronchi and bronchioles. Under normal conditions these cells secrete a thin layer of mucus and have small cilia on the surface which directs unwanted particles away from the lungs. When the cells are destroyed the body immediately produces new cells.

If small errors in cell structure (DNA) occur when they divide they can develop into cancer cells. These divide rapidly, which is characteristic of cancer cells. A cluster of such cancer cells is termed a *tumor*, and if these cells break through to the blood or lymph, they can spread to the entire body. In some places they will get stuck and continue the unrestrained cell division in what is called metastases.

Common symptoms of lung cancer are chronic coughing, phlegm with blood, impaired breathing, chest pains and weight loss. When the cancer is very advanced, there is probably not much an even perfect breathing can do to cure the disease. But soft and efficient breathing will give your body the maximum amount of oxygen. Moreover, the terrible feeling of not being able to breathe will to some extent be reduced. Removing the malignant tumor by radiotherapy can in some cases cure patients with lung cancer.

Alkaline blood caused by hyperventilation

When breathing becomes too fast or "nervous", also known as *hyperventilation*, large quantities of carbon dioxide are leached from your blood causing blood pH to rise to a more alkaline level (pH > 7,45). Symptoms range from dizziness, discomfort, fatigue, general irritation to headaches and chest pains. When the condition becomes more severe, you can experience a prickly, sticking or even burning sensation in the skin, particularly in the fingertips.

Hyperventilation is unfortunately self-reinforcing. The feeling of not being able to breathe is quite unpleasant, but you are actually receiving enough oxygen. The problem is that the body lacks carbon dioxide.

Luckily, this can easily be corrected by being conscious of your breath, especially of its frequency and depth. Breathe slowly and with control, hold your breath for 5-10 seconds after an inhalation then slowly exhale. When you hold your breath and/or exhale slowly, the carbon dioxide level in the body rises, and this is exactly what you want to achieve. Close your eyes and listen to your breath. You may also know the trick of breathing into a bag. This will also cause carbon dioxide levels to rise, but you are of course cheated of fresh air and thus oxygen!

Acidic blood caused by hypoventilation

If you breathe more slowly or weaker than usual, also called *hypoventilation*, the level of carbon dioxide in the blood rises. As a result of this, the amount of free hydrogen ions (H+) increases causing a increase in blood acidity (pH < 7,35). In very obese individuals a hypoventilatory syndrome can arise. Common symptoms are fatigue, confusion, drowsiness, shortness of breath, rapid exhaustion and in more acute cases unconsciousness. By creating a healthier and more efficient breath, preferably with some audible exhalations now and then, the acidity of the blood will become balanced because an appropriate amount of carbon dioxide leaves the blood through the lungs.

Holistic rehabilitation
- a case study

We have now looked at how breathing exercises and in some cases breath holding can be of potential help to patients suffering various diseases. Here is an example of how breathing exercises can be employed during treatment. It is a tangible illustration of how a more holistic approach can produce optimal results in the treatment of an illness.

In my opinion, a readily effective course of treatment can arise from the fusion of the old Asian wisdom, regarding the enormous impact that breathing can have on body and mind, with modern high-tech medical treatments and technical know-how such as sophisticated brain scans and genetic analysis.

When I teach efficient breathing to patients and students, we perform exercises on land as well as in water. Performing exercises in water has many advantages particularly for debilitated patients because it is easier to move in water, but they are naturally more laborious to set up. It is important that the exercises in water are always carried out under the supervision and guidance of a competent person who understands the various risks related to water workout. Don't forget – breath holding in water should never be performed on your own!

This case is a relatively detailed description of a treatment and rehabilitation progress following an acute illness. The patient suffered serious damage to the cerebellum caused by a tick bite that lead to a dramatic deterioration of his body over a period of time. The prospects were poor, but a marked improvement succeeded miraculously through holistic medicine and rehabilitation.

I hope that this example can provide useful information and shed light on a different and complementary form of rehabilitation and treatment. In the summer of 2007, my friend, Morten, had gone with some friends to a weekend cottage where they rode their mountain bikes into the woods. He removed a tick from above his right knee and gave it no further thought because as an active athlete he had removed many ticks before. A month later he received a rubella-like rash that covered his entire body and subsequently visited a doctor. The doctor thought the rash was just an inflammation similar to a throat infection and prescribed antibiotics.

The rash disappeared after a couple days, but he still felt strangely weak. As a genuine West Jutlander he did not fuss about it and thought the fatigue resulted from a busy life with two small children and a new job as human resource manager. Despite his weakened condition he travelled to France to work. During his presentations he repeatedly experienced sudden difficulties concentrating, which he had never experienced before. He also had trouble focusing visually, especially when he approached individuals and looked into their eyes.

This frightened him a bit, but he shrugged it off simply as possible symptoms of stress. After some days he was back in Denmark again, but he now felt so tired and uncomfortable that he could not go to work. He also suffered severe dizziness and had to lean on the walls when he moved about his apartment. Eventually it became so intense that Morten could no longer walk unaided, and he was hospitalized at Glostrup Hospital, Denmark.

Once he reached the hospital he was examined all over. The doctors took three samples of the fluid that surrounds the brain and spinal cord from his loin to analyze whether the bacterium *Borrelia*, found in ticks, was the cause. His symptoms suggested cancer of the lungs, so his lungs were X-rayed and his body and brain was scanned to locate a possible tumor.

After two days of tests the doctors tended towards multiple sclerosis as the most likely cause of Morten's symptoms. Subsequently, they started a treatment with corticosteroids which made Morten even weaker. At the hospital Morten's condition was continually getting worse. He was now fed antibiotics directly into his veins from a drip, had reduced mobility from the neck down and could not walk or stand. Three days after admission Morten was to have a new brain scan that would determine whether schlerosis was the cause. On his way over, a nurse came up to him and told him that the *Lyme disease* (*borreliosis*) test was positive. So it was a tick that had caused his illness. Morten's girlfriend, who was with him in the hospital, had never seen him so happy and relieved – partly because the cause now was determined and secondly, because schlerosis was ruled out.

Morten had been given antibiotics early in the course of treatment, though only a small amount. Several months had passed since the tick bit him and the *Borrelia bacteria* had subsequently spread to several areas of the brain including the cerebellum, which controls our coordination and equilibrium. Thus, he suffered the worst kind of Lyme disease which spread to the nervous system, called *neuroborreliosis*.

One of the main reasons that the doctors did not diagnose the disease immediately was that Morten had severe visual impairment, which had never been observed in a Lyme patient in Denmark. The bacteria had thus attacked the visual cortex just above the cerebellum. This explained his shifty glance, extreme dizziness and lack of balance.

When I spoke with Morten on the phone for the first time, I could hear that he had difficulties speaking, but it was still the good old Morten at the other end – with gallows humor and a sincere belief that he was "bloody going to walk again". And I totally agreed with him!

My first thought was that Morten should rehabilitate in water. Apart from the fact that water has an eminent "healing" power on the mind, the body is weightless and has an immense freedom of movement while the risk of overload injuries is almost eliminated. The natural resistance of water also trains the muscles differently than on land and the nervous system is greatly challenged at the same time.

My next thought was that he should learn some basic breathing exercises, which he could train in the hospital bed and during his balance training and workout.

I explained the key elements that he should be aware of during the exercises. Apart from focusing on being relaxed in his shoulders, neck and face, he should close his eyes. All breathing should be done through the nose, preferably with a hand on both his stomach and chest to become more familiar with a deep, controlled breath.

Furthermore, I tried to describe how he could perform *Victorious Breath*, but he could not quite find the right muscles in his neck and throat. I told him to just try it out, and that listening to his breath was the most important – with or without *Victorious Breath*.

Besides the serious equilibrium and coordination complications, Morten explained that one of the biggest problems he faced was to transfer from his bed to his wheelchair since he was very dizzy and shook so violently that the nurses were afraid they could not hold him. I remembered how "hook-breathing" in freediving helps by increasing oxygen tension in the lungs and stabilizes the body, and consequently suggested that he took a deep breath (through his nose) to oxygenate the body maximally and then – with full lungs – increase the air pressure in his lungs by tightening his diaphragm, abdominal, chest and neck muscles before the transfer to his wheelchair. This "trick" immediately proved to have a liberating effect. From then on, the transfers proceeded more smoothly, as his body was more stable, which allowed Morten and the staff to feel more safe. After a few days the transfer could be performed by just one assistant where two assistants had been required previously.

Morten left a voice message on my answering machine a few days later saying: "Hi Stiggy – it's Morten … we are talking 100% progress." I simply had to press "1" to listen to the message again. Yes, it was true – Morten was finally improving after four and a half weeks of inactivity.

I visited Morten at the hospital in Copenhagen a couple of days later to create a rehabilitation program and get him started with the exercises. I met Morten in the warm water pool in the basement of the Glostrup Hospital. It was wonderful to see him again, but at the same time shocking to find him confined to a wheelchair. His eyes were still shifty and his head was constantly shaking. The staff helped Morten to a hospital shower chair so that he could put his swimming trunks on. Then they placed him in a lift and transferred him to the pool.

We decided to divide the training into two major themes. The first focused on walking and equilibrium, and the second on swimming and diving. The general theme was obviously breathing, which was the focal point in all of the exercises.

Day 1, November 21st

Walking exercises were performed in deep water (approx. 160 cm) with a bar as support. The water thus supported most of the body and Morten could hold on to the bar – his balance was still too bad to walk unaided, and his whole body shook. We started off gently with the swimming part of the exercises, and I pulled Morten through the water while I supported his neck. When Morten felt comfortable, he tried to swim on his back – first using crawl legs, then breaststroke kicks, and both went amazingly well. Then he added his arms, and finally swam several lengths of crawl and breaststroke. I noticed that he was bothered with water entering his nose in both disciplines, and his technique was still lacking coordination, so I handed him my diving mask which instantly solved the problem. Towards the end of the session, Morten put a pair of flippers on and I asked him to swim a length underwater, which he did without hesitation.

"For the first time in five weeks I could do something without needing help. A feeling of freedom and the joy of being completely independent after receiving help 24 hours a day was beyond description. It was the beginning of a positive progression - I had not dared to dream that I would proceed so quickly."

Day 2, November 22nd

The following day we started with breathing exercises. Morten had practiced diligently and had become very good at breathing deep down into the "stomach". However, his stomach shook at the end of each inhalation, as his nerves in the lower portion of his body were affected the most. This imbalance around the abdomen and lower back hampered his progress and so we decided to direct more attention to this exercise. In addition, I introduced Morten to the *Brain Purification* exercise to allow him to strengthen and isolate the muscles in the abdomen and diaphragm and to clean the nose.

In the pool, Morten started with light "jogging" along the bar to warm up. Since his equilibrium was significantly better than the previous day, he went to the shallow part of the pool where a greater part of his body was above the surface. Here he was able to walk using a kickboard for support. After several strides back and forth, I took the kickboard from Morten and he walked on his own for the first time since admission.

"With a new awareness of my breath, calmness and stability was created that immediately made exercising easier, and it was the seed that lead to my first independent steps. My primary tools were *Victorious Breath* and deep "stomach" breathing. My focus had shifted from "having to walk" to concentrating on breathing in a new and different way which made a world of difference. When I focused too much on my walk, it all turned out messy. Somewhere deep inside my spine I was able to walk, so it was better to just let it happen naturally. The uniqueness of *Victorious Breath* was that it controlled my breath and in addition to being extremely soothing it stabilized the entire abdominal region because of the increased tension in the upper body."

We then came up with some mixed exercises like jumping with the legs together and walking sideways. Finally, we agreed that Morten should swim a crawl sprint, partly to work and train the muscles, and partly to challenge his heart and cardiovascular system. This was very difficult for him. In the meantime, one of Morten's physiotherapists (besides the one in the water) showed up, although she was off duty she had heard that "something exciting" was going on in the basement. Morten and I thought it was encouraging that she would spend her leisure time learning about new and different training methods.

Day 3, December 3rd

Morten stood with his crutches this time when I arrived at the warm water pool. He had been able to put his trunks on by himself, and it was a moving moment when he walked up the steel stairs to the pool. His movements were slow and his upper body shook a bit, but he managed on his own – without the help from others. Morten could now walk much better in the water. When he walked sideways his equilibrium was particularly good, even when he made large strides and put his legs together.

The physiotherapist suggested an exercise in which Morten should move a ball on the surface while turning from side to side, which would strengthen his abdominal and lateral muscles and challenge his equilibrium. Morten performed the exercise well, but gradually became very dizzy, as his eyes could not follow and kept jumping from side to side.

I thought Morten needed more focus on his breath in order to increase stability and make him calmer, and recalled that many of the yoga exercises coordinate a circular or a figure 8 motion with the breath. I thus developed a new exercise that, with a little fine-tuning, worked brilliantly. Morten started the exercise by holding the ball in front of him in outstretched arms, and when he moved the ball towards his chest he inhaled slowly. Then he slowly exhaled while he pushed the ball away from himself and at the same time started a circular movement to the right. When the ball reached an outer position (outstretched arms), he started to inhale again, as gently and harmoniously as the circular path that the ball drew in the water. The inhalation would be complete when the ball once more was in front of his chest.

Then the ball was led straight out during an exhalation, and the same circular movement repeated to the left side. Of course, *Victorious Breath* was used during the entire exercise, since the air resistance in the throat significantly contributes to a controlled breath. In addition, producing a sound has a positive effect on concentration and relaxation. Morten then performed a throwing and catching exercise and headed the ball to train eye coordination. A week before I joined Morten I had sent him a diving mask with a snorkel that attached in the front because his neck became stiff when he swam. The snorkel was an eminent tool that allowed him to swim with a relaxed neck not needing to turn his head to breathe. The mask avoided water from entering his nose. To put a bit of pressure on Morten, I asked him to swim eight lengths of interval training with the break between the lengths being shorter for every other length. He gave himself completely to the exercise and this concluded the day's water workout.

We then continued with the breathing exercises on land. The first exercise was pure "stomach" breathing, which went fine. Then I asked Morten to breathe only using his diaphragm, which was a big challenge for him. After a couple of minutes it went fairly well, but he had trouble isolating the diaphragm completely. The next exercise was the *Brain Purification* exercise, and now Morten showed improved strength, endurance and control. Finally, Morten practiced the *Victorious Breath*.

In the first phase the exhalation should be twice as long as the inhalation (a ratio of 1:2). This was an easy matter and Morten commented to me how amazingly fast this kind of breathing made him fully relax and gave him an immediate sense of peace and tranquillity.

The last phase was based on the classical pranayama yoga ratio of 1:4:2. Here, Morten held his breath between the inhalation and the exhalation, and this pause was four times as long as the inhalation. In the beginning I asked Morten to use his pulse to count (e.g. inhaling in four heartbeats, holding his breath during 16 heartbeats and finally exhaling during eight heartbeats). In the end, he also tried using the large clock that ticked loudly in the single ward. Both methods worked brilliantly.

After a rest and a lunch break, it was time for that day's walking exercise. Morten started off with the usual walk along the bar and when he had warmed up, he took his first independent steps on land without support. He used *Victorious Breath* throughout, but got tired when he forgot to focus on his breath. As soon as I made him aware of this, he regained his focus and proceeded with a more balanced and harmonious walk. Finally, he also walked sideways and challenged himself by constantly increasing the step-length.

> "When I performed my equilibrium exercises, it was crucial that I breathed deeply into the lungs using the diaphragm, since this enabled me to maintain my positions more safely and longer. I am convinced that it was one of the main factors that helped me back on my crutches again – at least a week earlier than it otherwise would have happened."

Day 4, December 7th

We began in the warm water and Morten started out with walking normally and then sideways. I asked Morten to perform skips, and he had no difficulties performing this exercise, which made the friendly care-staff smile (there should always be room for enjoyment). Next, Morten swam interval exercises wearing the diving mask and frontal snorkel, and when he was well warmed up I asked him to perform some dolphin leaps from the bottom. He made some forceful leaps, and when he subsequently performed high standing jumps, we could all see that Morten was regaining his original strength and equilibrium, which naturally was very motivating and encouraging.

To check Morten's balance, I asked him perform a yoga pose called the tree pose where you stand on one leg with your hands above your head. Morten focused on *Victorious Breath* and he stood surprisingly calm. Even when I asked him to close his eyes, he remained calm, which really impressed me, since this exercise is difficult even for healthy and well-trained people. Finally, we performed the ball exercise (*Victorious Breath* and figure 8 motion), and continued until the nice ladies at the poolside threw us out because some small children wanted to get in.

After a good lunch Morten practiced walking with his physiotherapist. Morten focused on coordinating the movements of the arms with the rest of the body. On an "obstacle course" (small rings and mats made of rubber to walk on) he was particularly aware of taking deep and calm breaths to maintain concentration. He then played a little soccer with the physiotherapist. Since Morten is crazy about soccer and is a former first league player, he was enthusiastic. It was like watching a little boy with a brand new bike - he was one big smile.

After this, I challenged Morten with some asanas. First, the so-called body-twist, followed by the shoulder stand and *Plough Pose*, which went well. Morten seemed particularly pleased with my self-invented variant of *Plough Pose*, where the knees are allowed to rest on your forehead. Then I showed the headstand to Morten, which he also wanted to try. However, this was a bit too much, and he became very dizzy and somewhat unwell, so I quickly helped him down from that position.

To conclude the program of that day, Morten did strength training with his shoulders, chest, back and legs all while focusing on breathing and holding his breath at high loads. Morten had completed all the exercises and walked around the rehabilitation room without his crutches.

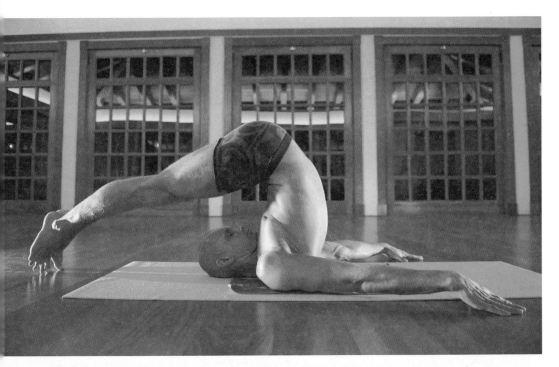

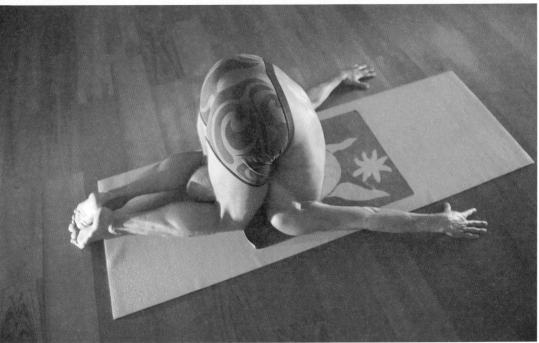

Plough Pose gives the body's internal organs a good massage. If the knees are lowered to the forehead or ears an extremely comforting and pleasant state of mind can be achieved.

Day 5, December 17th

I spoke with Morten on the phone and instructed him in *Alternate Nostril Breathing,* where the air changes direction in the nostrils during inhalation and exhalation. Morten told me that he had trouble keeping his equilibrium on a soft rubber plate in the morning, which the physiotherapist had asked him to train on, but as soon as he had focused entirely on a deep breath he had remained steadfast. The significant difference that the breath had on his performance impressed the physiotherapist, who said that she had never seen anything like it.

Day 6, January 11th

The anticipated day of Morten's discharge had finally arrived, but we still had to first go through the training program of the day. We mostly enjoyed just swimming about, but naturally Morten was not going to be let off lightly and the last exercise was a sprint interval where he swam faster and faster with shorter and shorter breaks between each lane. To make it even more challenging he swam a whole length underwater. To my surprise, and also to that of the physiotherapists present - who had played an important part of Morten's rehabilitation - I did not manage to run him tired. I mean really tired, exhausted.

In the subsequent workout on land, he showed great strength, coordination and equilibrium when he followed a line on the floor. Accordingly, Morten was ready for discharge and that afternoon we packed his things and waved goodbye to Glostrup Hospital, which had been a supportive home for almost four months. We threw Morten's luggage in the trunk of the car and headed for his apartment – "home, sweet home".

Morten has been to several follow-up consultations with both a specialist in eye diseases and a neurologist. His rehabilitation has been almost miraculous, and he continues to train on a daily basis to regain his functions completely. I will let Morten conclude and summarize the many long months that followed the tick bite he received in the woods and which changed his world in a second.

> "Remember, you have been in hell". Dan Milea, the doctor who examined my eyes said. The neurologist, Jesper Gyllenborg, who was there for me during the entire process, has since told me that he thought I would never walk again. Statements like these constantly

remind me how serious an illness I experienced. At the same time the experience has shown me how important it is to focus on new or different treatments.

As an athlete, it was important for me to be able to use my body while I was confined to the hospital. In particular the breathing exercises had helped me do something to actively relieve my situation. When you are used to managing everything, but suddenly find yourself 'dumped', it is fantastic to use the breath to make a difference.

The slow, deep and controlled breathing exercises provided me inner peace and a feeling of well-being that I could not obtain during the traumatic hospitalization. The challenging breathing exercises stimulated my nervous system and restored the contact between my nerves and muscles. Especially in the abdomen which shook uncontrollably. Specifically the little "hook-breathing" trick allowed me to manage the transfers from bed to wheelchair. This gave me freedom and made it possible for me to go to the toilet and bath on my own.

Throughout the rehabilitation process – the physical therapy and my workout – I focused on my breath and the mental stability and calmness it provided. It enabled me to constantly increase the challenge in the exercises and thus advance faster. It was clear to me that if for a moment I forgot to be conscious of my breath it would be difficult to perform even simple exercises.

In practice, this meant that within a few weeks I could perform relatively complex coordination, equilibrium and strengthening exercises that were beyond the level that we all hoped would be possible. The exercises in water proved absolutely wonderful for my recovery, because water supported my body and made it possible for me to perform exercises I could not perform on land. The first time we entered water I was actually quite concerned that I would roll over and lie like a dead person on the surface, but Stig's presence in the pool made me confident. Luckily, my concerns were unfounded, and I can recommend water exercises to different patient groups or people with work or sports injuries.

From working with my breathing I have discovered how little I actually know about myself and especially how my breathing affects me. As an athlete I know my body really well and I am familiar with its reactions and limitations, but today I realize that there is much to gain from a conscious breath when it is correctly applied to different situations. Although I have an MSc in sports and an MA in psychology and work as a human resource development manager, I believe that I have not given enough attention to the significance of the breath either during my education or in my everyday work to optimize the performance and work satisfaction of employees.

If my knowledge of breathing had been greater when I was an elite soccer player, I would surely have breathed more optimally e.g. when

I kicked penalties, free kicks or corner kicks. But I never thought about it. But what if I had done it differently and better? My team and I would have profited even more from it.

In the future I will use a conscious breath to optimize my own performance. I have learned that my breath can mediate inner peace that strengthens me, so why not use it in situations where I am under pressure or when I give presentations and need to be focused and sharp? It is also certain that I will incorporate breathing in a significant way in my work with coaching managers.

I am convinced that others can benefit from being focused on their breath when working as a manager. It can help a manager to be calm and present, which creates good performances. Actually, it is not only managers but everybody that should benefit from having knowledge and an awareness of their breath. In many everyday situations at home or at work your breath can be a friend that follows you and makes everything a bit easier and makes it feel right. In addition, it should be mentioned that the breath has a huge potential in healthcare. I have experienced this at close quarters.

Before I fell ill, I did not share Stig's interest in yoga and breathing exercises and was more focused on his technique, mental training, objectives and outcome. I actually thought that this "yoga stuff" sounded a bit strange, but now I know from personal experience that it is very effective, and has provided me with a much deeper and more nuanced understanding of myself as well as Stig's freediving universe and his preposterous and impressive records. I would like to thank Stig for that."

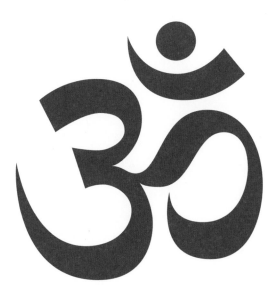

Exercises

1) CAT STRETCH

Start on all fours. Slowly breathe in while you arch your back like a cat and lower your head to look at your navel. Maintain the stretch 5-10 seconds and then breathe out while you sag your back and gaze at the ceiling. Repeat 10 times – arch and sag.

Perform the same exercise, but in a more dynamic and fast pace. Repeat 20 times.

In both exercises you can also try to "reverse" breathing – that is breathe out when you arch your back, and breathe in when you sag.

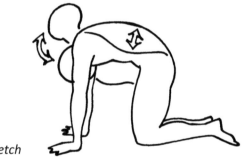

Cat stretch

2) WAG YOUR TAIL

Start on all fours. Keep your arms stretched and firmly fixed to the floor, so the body does not move. Slowly wag your back end to the side and forward, while you breathe in. Hold the position for 5-10 seconds. Then slowly breathe out and wag to the opposite side. Repeat 10 times from side to side.

In this exercise, you can also "reverse" breathing, and you can do it more dynamically. Remember to coordinate your breathing with your movements.

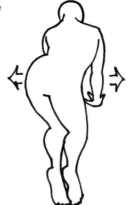

Wag your tail

3) RIGHT ANGLE

Lie on your back and lift your legs up to 90 degrees. You can place your hands beneath your buttocks for support. If this is not possible, then steady your legs up along a wall. Breathe quietly for 1-2 minutes.

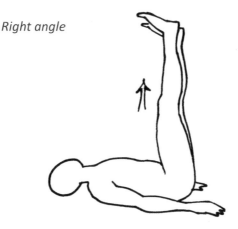

Right angle

4) PLOUGH POSE

Lie on your back and continue the exercise *Right Angle* by letting your knees fall towards you. Perhaps just to the chest, but preferably let the legs fall over you so that your toes hit the floor above your head, if possible. Beware, however, that the neck is okay throughout the exercise, because this exercise puts a lot of pressure on all the muscles in this area.

Possibly let your knees rest on your forehead, which immediately gives a soothing sensation. If you are very flexible you can drop your knees beside your ears. Hold the position for one - two minutes and continue to breathe calmly.

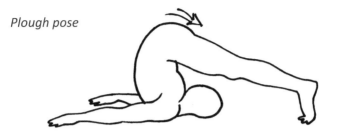

Plough pose

5) CHILD'S POSE

Rest on your knees and slowly bend over your thighs until you remain in a relaxed stooped posture. You can often rest your forehead on the floor in front of your knees. It does not matter if you cannot reach the floor with your forehead, and if necessary stack your hands on top of each other like two fists and rest your forehead on these to relax your neck and back. It is a pleasant and soothing feeling to sense a slight pressure on the forehead just above your nose – the third eye in the ajna chakra. Try it yourself!

Alternatively you can separate the knees slightly and let your torso rest between your thighs. Continue to breathe as naturally and calmly as possible.

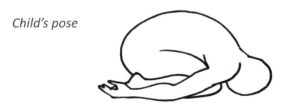

Child's pose

6) MAXIMUM EXHALATION

Lie on your back in *Relaxed Position*, but place your hands on your chest with your palms facing downwards. Breathe in through your nose and fill your lungs completely. Hold your breath for a couple of seconds and then breathe out as slowly as possible – either through the mouth or the nose. The exhalation may take anywhere from ten seconds to more than one minute. Keep exhaling until your lungs are completely empty.

Maximum exhalation

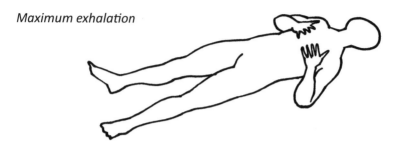

7) THE THREE LOCKS

Perform this exercise only after having completed a couple of exercises that warm up, stretch, and supple the lungs, chest and spine. Perform these locks (*Root Lock*, *Abdominal Lock* and *Throat Lock*) in a sitting posture when you practice breath holding in pranayama – e.g. in connection with *Victorious Breath* or *Alternate Nostril Breathing*. Besides having a strengthening and beneficial effect on your breath and your nervous system they also provide greater mental control.

1) *Root Lock*. Pull the muscles in the rectum and perineum together and hold it for 1-2 seconds in the beginning. The exercise is similar to the kegel exercises that many women perform to strengthen the pelvic floor. The exercise can be performed anywhere, whether you are watching television, attending a meeting, driving or working at your computer.

2) *Abdominal Lock*. This lock is called "*uddiyana*" in sanskrit, which means "flying up" or "being lifted". The lock is performed in connection with a breath hold on full or half full lungs and is performed by sucking your stomach and diaphragm inwards and upwards. In this way, not only the diaphragm "flies" but also your prana is directed upwards. This exercise is slightly more advanced than the little "swoop" you made in the exercise where you breathed with your diaphragm, and suction should be maintained for at least 5 seconds. Once your diaphragm is flexible and strong and your mental control determined, you will undoubtedly be able to hold the *Abdominal Lock* for one or several minutes.

3) *Throat Lock.* As previously described, *Throat Lock* is performed by closing your throat while pressing your chin down a bit and lifting your chest up. Like the Abdominal lock this exercise is performed when you hold your breath, and it holds the air in your lungs. One important thing to remember is that the *Throat Lock* has to be "unlocked" quietly before you breathe out!

Great Lock

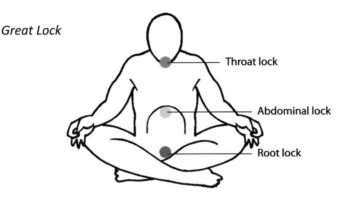

Throat lock

Abdominal lock

Root lock

Once you master these three locks, you can try to do them all at once in *Great Lock (Maha Bandha)*

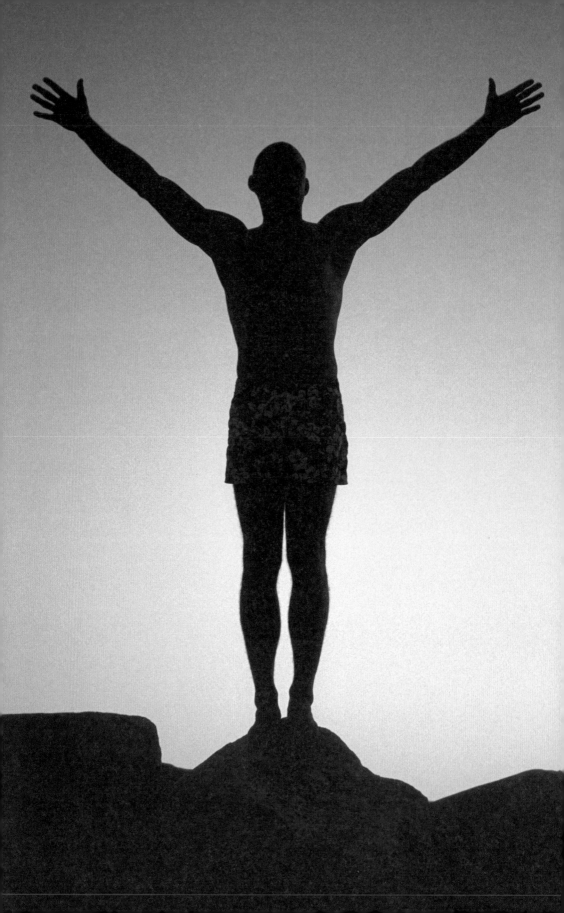

Soothing breathing

More pleasure less pain

Pain in body and mind

Chronic or passing pains are a daily problem for many people. Pain is often caused by disease, but can also be caused by overload, wear, or in connection with medication errors. A common treatment is painkillers - a treatment that relieves pain but does not eliminate the cause.

Recent studies have shown that over half of the adult population in the US use complementary or alternative medicine to supplement or replace their prescribed treatment. The same trend can be observed in Denmark and other European countries where there is an openness to a holistic approach. The most popular forms of alternative medicine in the body-mind category have been recommended by leading American authorities like the National Cancer Institute and the National Institute of Health, and in more recent years by the American Pain Association. This shows that a shift towards an holistic view of man is becoming permanent.

> "The mind is filled with luminous joy.
> He who practices pranayama is in truth happy."
>
> GHERANDA SAMHITA

Body-mind therapy focuses on the relationship between brain, mind, body and our behavior, and the combined effect of these components on our health and disease. Body-mind perception places great importance on cultivating and strengthening self-awareness and the ability to take care of oneself – two qualities that are key elements in yoga and freediving.

Relaxation exercises combined with breathing are commonly used in body-mind therapy, making it particularly effective against many stress-induced diseases. Other body-mind therapy techniques are meditation, yoga, hypnosis, imagery, biofeedback, tai chi and qi gong. Prayer and other spiritual rituals also belong to this group, but their precise impact is more difficult to evaluate.

In contrast, a growing body of scientific studies shows that breathing exercises and relaxation, often in combination with hypnosis or guided imagery, have a positive effect on pain. Accordingly, body-mind therapy has been used successfully in the treatment of ailments such as arthritis, chronic pains in the back and loin, headaches, migraines, ulcers and cancer.

The benefits of body-mind therapy are numerous. It is cheap to implement, highly safe, and above all easy to perform. The fact that patients with severe pain themselves are able to take an initiative and actively do something to relieve their pain has several secondary beneficial effects. For example, they feel more in control of their frustrating situation, and thus regain mental energy and spirit to live. The uniqueness of the breath in these cases is that it can be employed to varying extents depending on their condition.

Finally, it should be mentioned that it has been shown that pain before, during or after an operation is reduced when body-mind therapies are utilized, leading to a significant reduction or even elimination of medical anaesthetics.

How does body-mind therapy work?

There is a growing understanding of the underlying mechanisms of body-mind therapy. As described previously, thoughts can have a positive effect on the nervous system, hormone production and immune system.

> "A healthy mind in a healthy body."
>
> JUVENAL

A deep controlled breath is an obvious candidate for pain reduction, as it relaxes tense or cramped muscles and increases blood flow in the body, whereby cells acquire more oxygen and are cleansed of waste products. In addition, the mind is calmed by higher alpha wave activity in the brain; furthermore, the production of *endorphins*, the body's natural painkillers, is elevated. Increased amounts of endorphins are released when you are positive and happy, smile, kiss and especially when you laugh. But they can also be produced if you trick the body (and brain).

A recent study demonstrated the effect of placebo and the power of thought in a simple experiment where a number of subjects were administered a slight burning sensation to their forearm, after which a dummy ointment was smeared over the affected area. One half of the subjects were told that the ointment was pain-relieving. This made

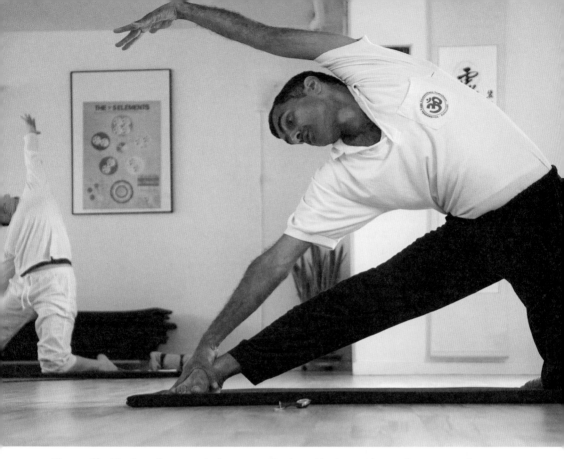

Yoga effectively relieves pain because the breath strengthens the connection between body and mind.

them produce endorphins naturally, which did not occur in the other group. This experiment shows the importance of what you believe, and not least what a therapist can make you believe. Similar studies have shown that care and trust in the therapist-patient relationship has a beneficial effect and emphasizes the complexity of the link between body and mind, but also its vulnerability. In short, it is vital to reassure and create a safe environment and particularly to convince the patients that a positive attitude makes a difference.

Furthermore, some very interesting brain scans have revealed that patients who have been anaesthetized by hypnosis exhibit less activity in the area of the brain where the pain is processed. In other words, pain is reduced. The initial pain signal transmitted e.g. from the skin, a muscle or a bone, however, remains unchanged, indicating that it is a change in the area of the brain where the pain is perceived that creates the analgesic effect.

"I lay myself down in the dentist's chair ready to have my cavity fixed. Aw, I didn't feel like lying there and having to spend the rest of the day at work with a half-stunned jaw, yes, I really don't feel like visiting the dentist at all and tried to postpone the visits as long as possible, but now I was here. My latest dental experience was six months ago and was associated with the memory of some pain. Now I was pregnant with my planned child and had refused anaesthesia during surgery because I feared of harming my child. The fear that something would harm my child was greater than the wish to spare myself the pain, so instead of avoiding the pain by a painkiller, I took the pain by the horns, so to speak, and counted down from 100 while I tried to breathe calmly into one nostril and out the other. I divided the countdown into intervals of 10, and at 46 I had to take a little break to wipe the tears away and collect myself a bit before we proceeded. Although I obviously wanted the pain to disappear, I never considered taking a painkiller, I knew the cause of the pain and knew why I exposed myself to this torment. It was, so to say, a conscious choice, and it made me feel that I could control it. It was not an enemy, just a necessary companion for a short time. For each interval we covered, I grew stronger and stronger, the pain received less and less attention and thus occupied less and less of my consciousness.

In the eyes of my new dentist this experience made me an individual with a "high pain threshold", and we ultimately decided to fix the cavity without any painkiller other than counting aloud and the aforementioned breathing exercise. My focus was on the counting and how strong and in control of the pain I felt for each completed interval: in a short period of time the drilling was over, and after a bit of polishing I returned to work without a hanging jaw and any feelings of inferiority that I as a 32-year old still get cavities in my teeth."

Sofie Ejlersen, MA Psychology, Process consultant and supervisor
In the dementia unit at Willow House, Denmark

Relieve pain mentally

Over 30 years ago, the American Professor Jon Kabat-Zinn initiated a series of experiments where mindfulness meditation and other yogic techniques were used to treat chronic pain. Mindfulness is an absorption in and acceptance of the present condition, and can be an easy tool to better manage pain.

You can also employ another strategy where you turn all your attention to something else – for example, through concentration – and thus create a distraction from the pain. The concept of flow is very important here. The Hungarian Professor of psychology, Mihaly Csikszentmihalyi, created the theory of flow in the early 1990s. It is based on being fully immersed in a perfect balance between challenges and skills where you can achieve a kind of comfortable, timeless and all-consuming state. The task you indulge in must therefore not be too easy nor too difficult. When someone reaches a perfect state of flow, the "normal" signals of the body are shut down and pain disappears completely. You may have heard about being "in the zone", which is the same as flow.

Personally, I believe that physical activity can help to catalyze the effect of flow. Therefore, I believe that people who suffer pain can greatly benefit from practicing sports that they are already interested in. The better you become at involving yourself and reaching a state of flow in your everyday life, the more endurable the pain will become – and the better it can be controlled.

I use both mindfulness and flow actively, particularly in connection with peak sports performances, where the pain sometimes reaches an unbearable level. As described earlier, during long dives lactic acid accumulates in my legs to such an extent that eventually I cannot move them. At the same time the diaphragm pumps vigorously up and down, and in general every cell in my body is crying out for oxygen. Sometimes I accept the pain as it is, while in other cases I "enter" the pain and examine it closer, and both strategies act as a kind of vigilant attention, as in mindfulness. I find it therapeutic and similar to the acceptance principle in ACT in the sense that the exercise of tolerating and accep-ting the pain during the breath hold can be transferred to other parts of my life. In the same way, others can benefit from this type of strategy where an accepting mindset can be used as a mental therapeutic tool to treat symptoms such as anxiety, fear, depression, obsessive compulsive disorder (OCD), post traumatic stress disorder (PTSD) and chronic pain.

When I reach a sufficiently challenged state, I pay no attention to the pain because I have reached "the other side" and have entered a state of flow. All my attention and consciousness merges with the activity I perform, and therefore no room is left to register or reflect on the pain. However, it is not always that easy to enter a state of flow because sometimes it hurts too much. The concentration and thought control fail me and I give up mentally. But if you train your mind, the intense pain becomes a kind of mental anchor or beacon that signals that pain will soon disappear. It is all about finding the right attitude. Once you have climbed the "mountain of pain", you can just sit back and enjoy the ride down.

A third strategy to optimize the body and mind's ability to relieve pain is by imagery. The more actively imagery is coupled with a controlled breath, the greater an effect it will have.

If you imagine that your body turns from blue to red, you may experience a warm sensation in your entire body. It is not purely imagination because your body can actually become warmer. The large muscles deep inside you and the muscles below your skin relax, blood circulation opens and internal heat is transported from the body core to the peripheral parts of your body.

Naturally, at the same time oxygen and nutrients are carried with the blood stream to the remote corners of your body and more waste products than usual are removed with the blood. In the same way nerves are calmed, and all of this helps you feel more fresh, relaxed, happy and positive. Pain diminishes, partly because of improved blood circulation, but also because the relaxed state leads to pain-relieving endorphins being directed to the entire body. Finally, deep relaxation also has a beneficial effect on the white blood cells - small soldiers in the body's immune system, which become better at fighting inflammations.

A wealth of different relaxation and imagery exercises exist, but you have to find the exercises that work best for you. As noted earlier, a calm and controlled breath will not only provide an immediate positive and calming effect at the physical level, but also strengthen the bridge to your subconscious mind and mental balance. In other words a proper breath will enable you to reach a relaxed and painless state faster.

Chronic pain in everyday life

Many people suffer daily from pain in different degrees. Whatever the cause of these pains, a common denominator is that they drain energy and happiness from everyday life. Luckily, pain often occurs in short periods, but in some instances it is chronic and can take up much of one's daily life.

Indeed, chronic pain can evolve and become a "natural" part of life, following like a little tormentor. Particularly with children this may become a big problem, because they often have difficulties defining the "pain" and do not regard it as something unnatural, but rather as something that presses, feels heavy, tightens or stings. Pain has many faces and comes in many shapes, but in order to relieve or eliminate pain, it is essential to find the cause.

Pain can be divided into several categories depending on their origin. In regards to physical damage on joints, muscles or bones as a result of work or sports injuries, pain-relieving medication is often the first treatment, after which comes rest and rehabilitation. When the cause is physical overload, the pain will usually disappear when the injury has healed. The breath is a clear and powerful tool to create a high level of relaxation and blood circulation during a healing or rehabilitation program, and can be useful in conjunction with treatments such as physiotherapy or chiropractition.

The number of work-related injuries such as "mouse arm", tensions in the neck or shoulders, and back injuries has grown markedly in recent years, which is why this area deserves considerable vigilance.

With regard to pain caused by poor working positions – or many repetitive moments – these have a huge negative impact on a person's activity at work and at home which is costly on many levels. Yet, to a great extent, these pains can be prevented or avoided by simple changes in one's habits and in one's environment. No human being is designed to spend six to twelve hours a day sitting bent over a computer screen and certainly not in a crouched position. It is no wonder that so many people suffer headaches, migraines, neck tensions and soreness in the shoulders, back and loin when the upper body is cramped in a fixed position for hours without a break day in and day out. This combined with mental stress (due to a busy and variable work schedule) makes matters even worse.

By becoming more aware of how your breath works in your everyday life and by sitting more erect in your chair and opening up your chest, many of the pains caused by poor working positions can be reduced. You can also ask your boss for a new and better office chair or an elevating desk to enable you to work standing up. You can even bring your own training ball (large rubber exercise ball) to work and sit on it. There are many advantages using the training ball including muscle and nerve stimulation in the back. Since there is no support for the back you will find yourself sitting in a much more erect and upright position that requires balance and in turn allows for a deeper and more efficient breathing. I strongly support the use of these training balls and have been happy to give them away to my family, friends and even colleagues at my previous job at the University of Aarhus. They are by far the best $30 that you, as a private person or employer, can invest in improving health, and I hope and believe that these training balls will become more widespread in the future. These fun training balls are also an excellent tool for rehabilitation and for training strength, endurance and flexibility.

Many small damages and pains like the "mouse arm", *tenosynovitis* of the forearm or more serious complications in the shoulders and loin can also be eliminated by changing the monotonous physical routine. In the long run, many repetitive movements will severely wear the body down so a greater body awareness and an ability to create new solutions can be extremely beneficial.

Muscle tensions in the neck and back can also be effectively remedied by performing 10-20 deep and calm breaths while the shoulders are lifted and lowered. A brief walk in fresh air, preferably combined with a few simple stretching exercises, can also make tension and pain disappear, and indeed it is food for thought that such simple methods can improve your everyday life. To a large extent it is a matter of changing habits and attitude – both in yourself and in your boss.

Pain in severe illness

Temporary or incurable illnesses are often, to a greater or lesser degree, accompanied by pain. In order to mitigate severe pain, opioid therapy is often employed, which is a medical treatment using e.g. morphine, methadone, ketogan or codein. These drugs are certainly effective, but the problem is their potential adverse side-effects such as addiction, mood swings, lethargy and respiratory problems.

However, there are several examples where body-mind therapies have proven to be very effective, even in the case of serious diseases. For example, a group of patients with chronic pain in the back showed that a 12-week yoga program provided better results than 12-weeks of physical training or education. Likewise, various breathing and relaxation techniques helped pains in the back. A 10-week program based on mindfulness meditation has also shown a significant short and long term reduction in the degree of pain. Overall, this confirms that various body-mind therapies may be combined usefully with traditional medical treatment.

In relation to chronic pain, mindfulness has the advantage that you adopt a non-judgmental acceptance of the current situation and thus work with your pain instead of against it. When a person with pain is instructed, trained and supported in taking responsibility for his or her own situation, the pain will no longer be a factor that has to be overcome, but rather a teacher or guide into the relationship between body and mind.

You could also consider using body-mind therapy before a medical treatment is initiated. It will be interesting to see the extent to which this kind of therapy can reduce the use of pain relieving drugs.

However, there is the "problem", or rather a challenge with most of the body-mind treatments, in which the beneficial effects only become clear after prolonged use and adaptation. In a time when many people expect to lose weight by simply eating a little magic pill and do not consider changing either their diet or exercise habits, it can be difficult to involve palliative or curative methods that require commitment, time and energy.

Luckily, a controlled and calm breath does not only provide results over the long-term, but also a direct bonus in the form of a lower respiratory rate, lowered pulse and blood pressure and a higher degree of relaxation, so it will always be a good place to start.

Psychosomatic pains

According to holistic philosophy our pain and illnesses are caused by the sum of our mental and body processes. In other words, we are talking about an interaction that does not regard pain as an isolated bodily or mental problem, but rather an imbalance in the system.

In psychology, patients with chronic pain are helped by starting from the patient's own experiences and life situation. The hypothesis is that personal interpretations, traumatic events and daily stress leave permanent traces in the body, because it has its own "intelligence". These traces, which are the body's own counter reaction to all the events it has been through, whether you recall them or not, can be expressed as illness, headaches, muscle tension, spontaneous or unconscious breath holding pauses, stiff or impaired movement and of course as temporary or chronic pain.

By creating awareness among patients about how these things arise and develop as a result of personal feelings, attitudes, habits and body patterns, it is possible to work with them and ultimately make the pain go away. When a person sees his or her own life story in a new light, a spontaneous desire to create change appears along with the intention to eliminate the cause of the pain.

It is exactly the same point I start from when I give courses in stress management and efficient breathing, but instead of stories I closely observe the "intelligent" body language and its habits. The participants try both breath holding and forceful breathing, which I have experienced as very efficient tools for personal development. When I do sessions with "underwater meditation" where people do breath holding and learn different relaxation, imagery and concentration techniques, the participants get in contact with themselves in a completely new way, which penetrates right down to the cellular level. This is so because breath holding creates a good foundation for a different and intense way of experiencing and meeting yourself in body, mind and soul.

Unlike a psychologist, I cannot cure patients simply by talking to them. I cannot create change in a person who does not want it, but I can help inspire self-help.

However, it is very important for me to point out that it is not always a pleasant, much less easy and painless process to work with yourself. Self-insight requires that you work hard on both the light side and the dark side of yourself. You have to dare to grasp those rattling skeletons that you would rather not think about or that you have forgotten!

This kind of introspective meditation, which is an inner journey through your conscious and subconscious mind often moves back in time and can therefore be transcendent and shocking. Meditation is not merely pink elephants, dancing suns and warm light, but also a passage into the deeper layers of the mind, which is not always easy or pleasant to deal with.

I am often told that I "push" people. It is certainly true, but I never push people beyond the mental and physical point that I consider safe. But I like to push hard to help open new doors for self-development, because I cannot create change, only offer the possibility. Whether I work with bank directors, elite swimmers, disabled or just completely "ordinary" people, I do it the same way. Then people can do with it what they want. Here we reach the extremes, because as in yoga, freediving, medical science, business and everything else in life, it is in the border area that great changes take place.

Bedridden patients

All bedridden patients have plenty of time available and it is a privilege that should be fully exploited. Naturally, it can seem boring, futile and downright horrible to constantly lie in bed, but there are many activities that can be pain relieving to keep you occupied. It is also important to

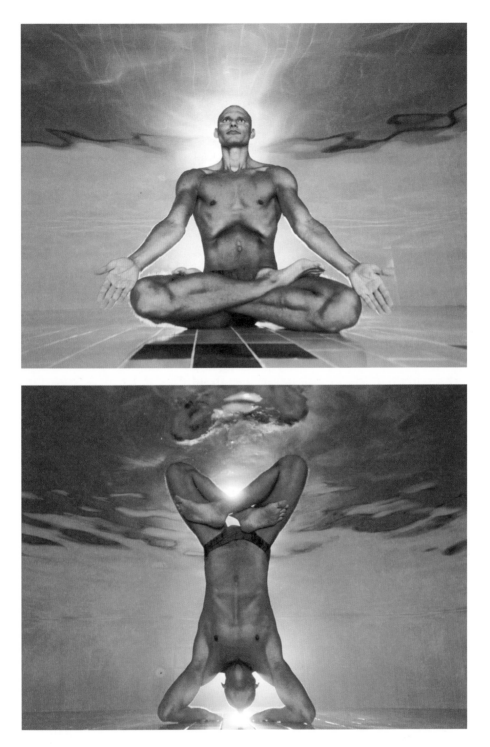

Our consciousness enables us to perform prolonged breath holds - if we want to - thereby calming our nervous system.

be aware of the fact that being motionless is unnatural for the body, which thus does not get its daily dose of exercise.

In this context the breath is a delightful companion, because you can train your breathing anywhere and anytime. As previously described, various breathing exercises help to keep your body in good physical shape and cleanse the entire system. With your breath you always have a calming and pain-relieving remedy at hand. For instance, patients with burns, cancer or other serious ailments often use deep and calm breaths in combination with relaxation exercises. If you are bedridden due to a broken leg, surgery, or even less serious injuries, you can still experience severe pain, and it is therefore advantageous to be able to distract yourself from it.

It is also worthwhile to be inspired by positive psychology, for example using mindfulness and flow, as these have the potential to produce a bright and optimistic way of thinking. Through a positive internal dialogue, the healing process is promoted. Mind training can be very helpful to patients who experience extreme pain or are very disabled, since it both relieves pain and increases mobility. The clever thing is that the brain cannot distinguish whether the movement actually occurred in the real world or only in the mind. The effect is a strengthening of the muscle-nerve connections and the body's general condition is improved.

Mindfulness meditation teaches you to accept the fact that you are confined to a bed. I also believe that getting into a state of flow is a strong pain-relieving tool for bedridden patients, whether they have slight or severe pain. The trick is to find the activities and creative pursuits a person can lose him or herself completely in – be it drawing, playing, listening to music, doing puzzles or something else.

Flow is typically characterized by a sense of timelessness while engaging in an activity that is meaningful and challenging. It can activate play-like emotions and moods, devotion, joy, pleasure, ecstasy, absorption, lightness, full presence, self-forgetfulness, enthusiasm, personal control and pride as some of the key concepts. Flow strengthens identity and self-esteem, and in repressing the self-consciousness the feeling of pain also disappears.

We have also looked at how a well-trained breath can be strengthened and may subconsciously act as a mental anchor that arouses special inner feelings. I also believe that a well-regulated and calm breath can assist in increasing the possibility of reaching a state of flow during creative activities – first through a conscious and controlled breath, and eventually through an unconscious breath.

Pain in elderly

Several studies have established that older people respond as well as (or even better than) young people to pain treatment through body-mind therapy. Previously, this has not been the general opinion because cognitive therapies in particular have been considered to be over-challenging to the elderly. However, they are not often offered these therapies and because many older people do not want to be a burden or ask for help, they are rarely given them, which is a shame.

Since elderly people often suffer from a number of diseases or disabilities simultaneously causing daily pain, many of them receive pain-relieving medication. However, elderly people can only tolerate the medication in small doses, and because they often have to receive it for the rest of their lives, it would be desirable to have a good and safe alternative to pain-relieving medication. Since almost every fifth person in the Nordic countries dies as a result of medication errors, this is also a strong argument for reducing the daily dose as much as possible. The group of elderly is growing steadily as well because today people live longer, so the more active and pain-free life you can lead, the better.

One of the biggest problems that elderly people face is that their pain or restricted mobility often prevents them from participating in social activities, thus they often become isolated, which can potentially lead to depression. It is a vicious spiral that can bring them down mentally, which in turn may increase the level of real pain as well as the focus on it.

For the elderly to feel that they can do something to affect the pain is often the first step in the right direction. A positive mind, extroversion and engagement in social activities will automatically lead to a healthier and more mobile body, and the positive effects, like a strengthened immune system and higher energy levels, will follow. An improved immune system will not only keep diseases at bay, but also reduce the natural aging process and increase the healing of sores or inflammation.

As an example I will refer to my father, who is 74 and suffers pain in the hip and lower back, despite the fact that he is otherwise very youthful, strong and active. Every morning he practices 20 - 30 minutes of workout on a training ball (the aforementioned large rubber ball), which I gave to him several years ago. His morning workouts consist of a series of exercises that focus on stretching, relaxation, endurance and breathing. If he skips the exercises for just a day or two, his pain immediately increases, so apart from the fact that he likes to stay fit, the pain relief from training also provides a good incentive to keep going.

It can be an advantage to bring body-mind therapy into the daily life or pain treatment of patients, because the more you learn how to activate the body's own medicine, the less medication you will need and the higher quality of life you will experience.

As mentioned earlier, base-forming foods have been used in the treatment of e.g. arthritis and back pain. So it is quite significant to your body what you choose to gorge yourself on, because whether you are young or elderly, it has a major impact on both your body and mind. How you decide to live your life is entirely up to you, but it is actually not a huge sacrifice or effort to choose a "live strong – die old" philosophy. If you eat healthier, your body will work optimally, and the reward will be that you feel better in your daily life and thus live longer and healthier. You should avoid eating too many sweets and fatty foods, eat more vegetables and base-forming foods, exercise regularly, smile, think positive and remember to breathe.

"After several months with an increased stress level, I could sense "electrical" shocks in my stomach when everything was at boiling point. I went to the hospital several times to make it calm down, but I looked for a better solution than painkillers and tranquilizers. I consulted Stig and explained the situation to him, and together we created a program with simple breathing exercises that I could perform anywhere – in the car, at work and in my bed – to be better at relaxing. Then I began to use the exercises and still practice them if there is pressure at work or I feel pain. It only takes a few minutes and helps to relieve my tension immensely.

However, the most important thing that made me change the way I perceive my body was the following sentence: "You have to listen to your body. No one knows your body better than you do."

Earlier I lived my life and the body just had to follow. Now I listen to my body in everything I do. At the same time I have become more disciplined with regards to my diet and exercise."

Thomas Dubosc, 35
Branch Manager at Transfer International, Le Havre, France

Stress release during pregnancy

As described the breath can relieve pain and help shift your focus. If you use your energy on breathing effectively, you will also spend less energy on pain, which then loses its intensity. This is common knowledge among midwives, who instruct pregnant women to use their breath as a tool to resist powerful contractions during labor.

A woman will feel some of the most intense pains in her life during childbirth. A majority of the mothers who give birth for the first time, describe the pains as severe or intolerable, whereas women, who have given birth several times experience the pain less severely each consecutive time.

The pain in women who have given birth for either the first or successive times are probably equally severe; but since the latter group has done it before, they know what to expect, can manage the situation better, and the birth usually proceeds faster. Hence, they often avoid severe or prolonged pain caused by fatigue or other complications.

This is interesting and indicates that a better understanding of the expected pain, the events occurring and the tools to better manage the stress in connection with childbirth can help to alleviate the experienced pain. The breath and the mental attitude deserve serious attention in this context.

Women can experience both mental and physical stress during pregnancy and birth. The breath can be used to manage this stress, which will benefit both mother and child.

As mentioned, stress is often caused by uncertainty or even fear of something unknown or different. Mental stress is independent of whether the "threat" is real or not, and this stress will often lead to undesired physical changes in the body. This in turn will lead to further anxiety, lethargy or weariness, as well as different symptoms such as an elevated pulse, hypertension, headache or sleeping disorders.

In addition to the mental stress a real physical stress and pain appears, which is the natural consequence of the many changes occurring in the pregnant woman's body, and increasingly so during the actual birth where the female body is exposed to extreme strain.

Because the fetus senses the mother's pulse and is in direct contact with her circulatory system, it is obviously important to eat healthy and workout, in order to give the child the best possible developmental opportunities. Excessively high levels of sugar and fat in the maternal blood is undesirable, and a high concentration of sugar may in fact lead to diabetes during pregnancy, which in turn affects child development negatively. If the heart rate or blood pressure is constantly too high, because of stress for example, this may also affect the fetus. Although it may seem a bit illogical, a state of hypertension can actually reduce blood flow to the placenta, resulting in a low birth weight infant who has received reduced oxygen and thus is stressed physically.

A number of clinical studies have shown that stress, nervousness and anxiety during pregnancy and childbirth are among the factors affecting mother and child the most. It has even been shown that women who are highly stressed during pregnancy are also at greater risk of developing post-natal depression.

As mentioned in connection with stress management, stress is regulated by two very complex systems that have a major impact on the body. Experiments on gravid rats have shown that stress not only changes the mother's but also the offspring's ability to manage stress. In the mother, stress affects the cortisol producing system and this is passed on to the young, which is born with a system that is permanently changed and consequently extremely sensitive to stress. These studies are not only interesting but also scary in the sense that the mother's stress is inherited by her young – not genetically but socio-physiologically. In other words, female offspring will in the future have a tendency to give birth to stressed offspring.

What we are talking about is a negative environmental spiral that spins downward very quickly, and that might explain a part of the dramatic increase in stress, as seen in children and adolescents today. If you as a future mother would like to break this spiral, one of the best things you can do is to breathe consciously and with control. In this way, not only the mother's stress system is toned down, but also that which is passed to the child. One of the most important factors for a pregnant woman to consider is to work on relaxing and managing stress, and in this context various body-mind strategies can be a beneficial addition to the established pregnancy and childbirth preparations. Despite the well-documented link between maternal stress and child development, very few studies exist to demonstrate the potential that various forms of body-mind therapy may offer pregnant and laboring women. Both yoga and meditation can be extremely beneficial during pregnancy and birth, and both can result in higher birth weight, a shorter period of pregnancy and birth, fewer instrumental interventions during labor, and reduced pain and tension.

Before birth

Flexibility exercises for the upper body and constant nose breathing are important to a future mother. The better the breathing, the more oxygenated and cleansed the body of the mother and in turn, the child will be. The symptoms of an ineffective maternal breath will often include dizziness, fatigue or headache, whereas a good and controlled breath will supply energy, calmness and a deeper, more sound sleep.

Deep and controlled breaths in combination with imagery exercises that enhance your self-esteem and feelings of joy will also increase the level of endorphins and decrease the pain of pregnancy and childbirth. Practicing kegel exercises (eg. *Root Lock*), is also something that is essential in preparing pregnant women for childbirth, as it strengthens the pelvic floor. It can be used to recover from childbirth as well.

Over the past three decades, in several Scandinavian countries the official health care policy has been that every pregnant woman has a right to effective pain management. There has been an increase in the use of medical pain relief by local anaesthetic, nitrous oxide or epidural anaesthesia but a neglect of natural pain reliefs such as acupuncture, baths, subcutaneous water injections, massage etc.

Concurrently, traditional and natural pregnancy and prenatal courses, which were very prevalent throughout the 1970s and 1980s, have been pushed aside, often for cost savings. In addition, restructuring and downsizing has lead to less time and fewer hands in many hospitals resulting in pregnant women not always receiving the proper information and practical knowledge they need during pregnancy and labor.

It is important that the pregnant woman gains self-awareness in relation to birth, so that she can behave rationally, calmly, accepting and "mindful" – especially with regard to pain.

Fortunately, I am happy to say that a greater interest in the ancient Asian techniques, which are based on the whole person and his/her environment, is emerging – or perhaps rather re-emerging. Hopefully there will be a greater focus on the pregnant women's needs. You can now be assigned to a *"doula"*, a professional person who is trained to help and advise women during pregnancy and childbirth. The term "doula" comes from Greek meaning "a woman who serves" and the trend comes from the US. For many years now, it has also been made possible to have a doula assigned to pregnant women in Scandinavian countries such as Norway and Sweden - however, the education of doulas was first initiated in Denmark in 2005.

Every doula has given birth herself and can help during pregnancy and childbirth and even after birth. A major advantage of a doula is that she does not help with the medical part of the birth, which is entirely left to the midwife, doctor and nurse, so she can fully concentrate on gui-

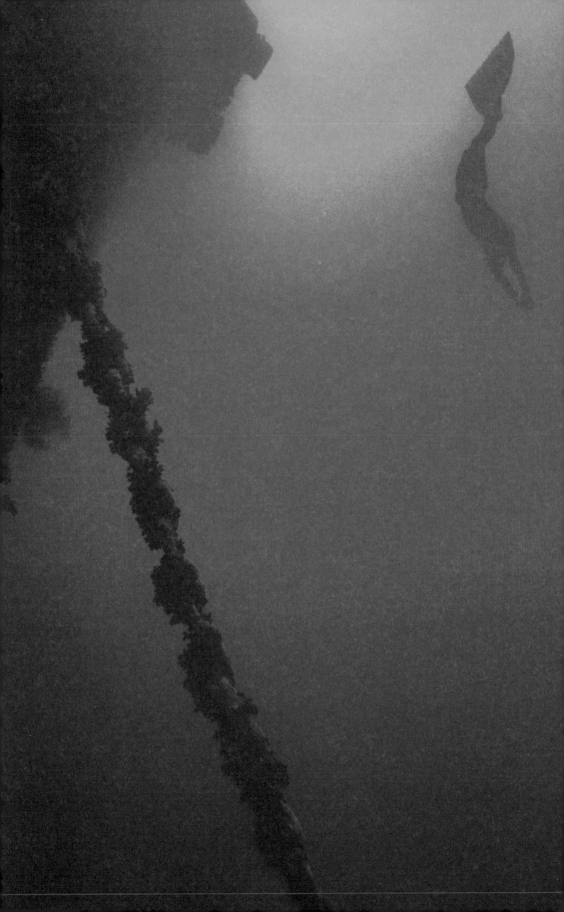

The pleasant and timeless state flow can be experienced during physical activity or during quiet but complete absorption.

ding and mentoring the laboring woman and perhaps her partner. Her help consists of offering emotional support, directly helping the woman to assume advantageous positions, giving massage or instructing her to perform simple breathing exercises - and of course just being present.

It is a great idea to have a professional and competent person assigned to you who can assist during the entire pregnancy process and create security and peace. It has been documented that the effect of having a doula present results in having a shorter birth process, less pain and fewer birth interventions – collectively called the "doula effect". In concrete figures the number of caesarean sections are reduced by nearly 50% and the consumption of pain-relieving drugs and medical labor induction are reduced by 30% and 40% respectively.

It is not surprising that a thorough preparation during pregnancy gives rise to the best possible birth experiences, and emphasizes the importance of the pregnant woman being physically and mentally prepared. Since not everyone has the opportunity to pay for private help or wants a stranger to participate during the birth, there are other possibilities. It would be equally beneficial for the pregnant woman to participate in yoga classes or relaxation training, strengthening her abdominal muscles and diaphragm and to engage in birth groups or other activities. It is often a good idea if the partner likewise participates in some of these exercises.

During birth

Whether a pregnant woman has used yoga or breathing exercises to prepare herself or not, the midwife will focus on the breath during childbirth. In other countries, where the pain-relieving treatments that are offered in Denmark are not readily available, the breath is often the strongest way to ensure a successful birth and relieve pain.

A well-regulated and calm breathing can create a more peaceful experience and bestow a greater sense of control and thus have a definite pain-relieving effect regarding the contractions, which a woman in labor will experience as less severe if she is not worried or tense. Just as when I hold my breath for five-six minutes, and my diaphragmatic contractions persist, labor pains also persist even after good breathing. But by becoming aware of them, accepting them and using the breath to gain mental control, they can be made more soft and comfortable.

It is also important that the laboring woman breathes through her nose because as we have previously seen, the blood is significantly better oxygenated in this way. Whether air is exhaled through the nose or mouth is of little importance. Nose breathing will also be key if the fetal heart beat changes, or in the instances that extra oxygen from a mask is needed.

Several different breathing techniques are employed during childbirth. One method is to hold your breath for a moment after inhalation before you exhale again. In this way you avoid hyperventilating and the blood is oxygenated more effectively and you avoid dizziness.

Another technique can be employed when the woman has the urge to push during labor and has to withhold the push just before the child's head is to be born. This technique is used to prevent the woman from pushing inappropriately, as this can damage the mother as well as the child. The technique can either consist of "gasping" breaths where the woman breathes in small fast intervals, or by a slow and controlled exhalation. Both types of breathing prevent the woman from pushing with full force.

In contrast she can push much harder when her lungs are full, because her loin, abdomen and diaphragm can exercise a greater pressure, similar to when we have to lift or move something heavy. You could say that this kind of restrained breath is hook-breathing, which oxygenates the body maximally, while lending support and strength.

In the midwife profession this is called the Valsalva method. The laboring woman is instructed to take a deep breath when her labor pains begin and then hold her breath as long as she can while she pushes. Then she should exhale and quickly inhale to push again. During a labor pain she should push two-three times. Since this is the most effective method it is often used for first-time mothers where the pushing period may be longer due to tight muscles in the pelvic floor. The method is also excellent if the laboring woman finds it difficult to push or if the child needs to be delivered quickly because of a poor heartbeat.

A slightly different method is the so-called "spontaneous pushing" technique, where the woman is allowed to push whenever she feels like it. In other words she breathes naturally and pushes when she feels the urge to while maintaining the push as long as necessary. This often results in shorter and more frequent pushes. Nonetheless, this method can be beneficial because the laboring woman holds her breath for a shorter period of time, thereby affecting the child's heartbeat less. For some women this method is also more comfortable but unfortunately it is not as effective and is almost exclusively used by experienced mothers who tend to have an easier and faster birth.

When considering all of the benefits, it is clear that the breath is an obvious and powerful tool during pregnancy and childbirth to ensure a healthy development of the child. Although the breath plays a central role in this context today, its enormous potential should be explored and utilized to a greater extent in the future. Not only is it free, simple and accessible to everybody, but it also provides formidable opportunities for a successful birth with few, or in some cases no pain relieving drugs. This may seem desirable for a future mother, who wishes to give birth in the most natural way.

If it is possible for women to give birth without any pain relief, the possibility of harm being inflicted on mother and child during intervention is reduced. The pregnant woman can move more freely and naturally, and at the same time she wins an enormous personal victory. This also has the potential to lead to a stronger sense of self-confidence and more energy to manage her newfound motherhood.

Breathing and relaxation exercises in water should also be employed more proactively. In this marvellous element the pregnant woman can relax more easily and deeply than on land due to the weightlessness. It is also easier to find a comfortable resting position, which can act both calming and relieving. In fact, the "magical" properties of water should receive much more attention in any kind of relaxation, de-stress and pain relief.

Hopefully the concept of breatheology and the exercises presented in this book have given you some practical and easy-to-use tools for your everyday life. You can find more information in our international community where you can also get free breathing tutorial videos. Visit www. breatheology.com and share your thoughts and experiences.

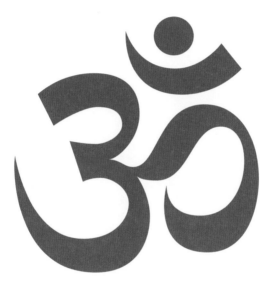

Exercises

If you suffer pain such as headaches, sore muscles or are dealing with a serious illness, the following exercises may have a soothing effect. Remember the inner (and if possible outer) smile, and laugh as often as you can – even at pain!

Breathe in through your nose and breathe out through your nose or mouth as you please.

If you do not feel that the exercises have an effect the first time you perform them, do not give up but try again on another day. The more you practice, the better you will be at strengthening the connection between body and mind.

1) Gently breathe out and focus on the sore or painful area, while one hand (yours or someone else's) touches the area. In this way you achieve maximum awareness and can loosen up e.g. cramped muscles in the neck or shoulders. When you consciously "let go" of the area through nerve impulses from the brain, the muscles release their cramped condition. You can clearly feel the muscle "letting go" – like when you stretch a tense calf after a long run.

2) Gently breathe out and focus your consciousness on your breath. Press your lips together or hold the air back with your tongue to produce a "pseeeee" sound when you breathe out. Now visualize the place where you experienced pain, and imagine that the area heals more and more for each exhalation. Feel the heat spreading in precisely the areas that you focus on. This exercise can easily take 5-10 minutes.

3) Try hyperventilating energetically with 10-20 breaths. This breathing pattern often occurs spontaneously in laboring women and in people who experience sudden pain. Readily produce an audible sound and concentrate solely on the breathing mechanism. An intense hyperventilation will lead to many temporary changes in your body – your blood pressure will rise, your heart will work faster, the acidity of your blood will change and you will secrete a lot of adrenalin, which "prepares you for battle". With all these distractions, you are bound to redirect your focus from the pain. It will become secondary to the many other changes that occur in your body.

4) Do 10 hook breaths by pushing the diaphragm and chest down after a full inhalation. You probably use hook breathing spontaneously when you lift something heavy. This is also used by laboring women. In this way you create a higher oxygen tension in your lungs, which will lead to a greater oxygen concentration in the blood. Apart from temporarily changing your oxygen tension and blood pressure, it will also stimulate your nerves and create a kind of relaxation afterwards.

5) Take a walk in a forest, find a deserted beach or lie down under your comforter. Scream at the top of your lungs. Do it 5-10 times. This will loosen up physical and mental tension, frustration and pain. By freeing yourself and stimulating your lungs, diaphragm, solar plexus and the rest of your nervous system, you create a soothing and refreshing sensation throughout your body. This is also a good exercise to use when you have stress.

6) Breathe calmly – use *Victorious Breath*, if you like. Make your exhalation twice as long as your inhalation as in the simple pranayama exercises, as this will have a strong stimulatory effect on your vagus nerve and thus the entire soothing part of the nervous system. At the same time, try to "enter" the pain. Examine it and accept it. In time you will become so eager to "investigate" your pain that it will disappear completely.

7) Breathe calmly using the Victorious breath and take as much time as you can breathing out. Exhale through the mouth instead of the nose, and produce a deep and soft "hmmmmmmmm" sound. You can also make it sharper and higher "heeeeeee", if you feel like it. The sound should be as smooth and melodic as possible. This is a pranayama exercise and is called *bhramari*. In Sanskrit *bhramara* means "bumblebee", so this is the sound you should try to imitate. The exercise creates a lot of vibrations throughout your body and vitalizes your cells with a micro-massage. Apart from cleansing your cells and your nervous system, bhramari is also a formidable relaxation and concentration exercise that is good for *insomnia*. Alternatively, use the sacred mantra Om (pronounced "AAAAUUUMMMMMM"). This mantra is sure to make you feel the vitalizing vibrations in your entire body, at first in your chest and then your throat, jaws and your head. Besides oxygenating your lungs and having a relaxing and de-stressing effect, it will prepare you mentally to accept and cope with your pain.

8) Perform the exercise *Paradise* and use all your senses to experience the place as intensely as possible. Expand the exercise by observing

yourself moving around in your paradise, light as a feather and without any tension or pain. Make sure your breath is as smooth and effortless as your weightless walk. In time, you will also be able to lower the sensitivity in the area of the brain where pain impressions are processed, whereby the discomfort seems less severe.

Appendix

Lifesaving first aid

Cardio Pulmonary Resuscitation (CPR)

The lifesaving breath

When we breathe air is sucked into the lungs, and shortly after the heart pumps oxygen to every cell in the body. As for oxygen, your brain is naturally the most demanding organ – it uses up to 20% of your total oxygen consumption as you sit and read these lines, despite the fact that it only represents 2% of your total body weight. In addition to being the greatest consumer of oxygen in the body it is also the most sensitive to changes in oxygen level. If for some reason you are low on oxygen, the brain will be the first to suffer damage.

Now imagine the following scenario: It has been a lovely but busy day and you have just stopped by your local shopping center to buy some groceries. As you are waiting in the line, the elderly lady in front of you suddenly drops lifeless to the floor – what do you do? Although it is not a pleasant thought, try imagining that this is your best friend or a beloved family member. Yes, it could even be you! About 164,000 out-of-hospital cardiac arrests occur annually in the United States. Of these, only 27.4% receive bystander CPR (Cardio Pulmonary Resuscitation). The survival rate for out-of-hospital cardiac arrest is around 5%. This figure is far too low. Unfortunately, many do not survive because they do not receive proper CPR in time. This is extremely sad since an effective rescue operation is simple to perform and can double the probability of survival.

I have always wondered why CPR courses are not mandatory in school. Similarly, I have often wondered why people wouldn't spend a night or weekend taking a CPR course. It is actually surprisingly little that is needed to save another human being's life – CPR is not a sophisticated operation.

Over the years, I have attended several diving and lifeguard courses where CPR was taught. I have also studied relevant websites, taken additional courses at the Danish Emergency Management Agency and updated my knowledge about the latest guidelines at an advanced course in Sweden. Furthermore, I have spoken with doctors and coast lifeguards who are very competent in this field.

The courses are easy to pass and inexpensive. CPR courses are offered everywhere and you generally become well-prepared at managing a situation where someone is in distress. It is nice to know that you can help make a difference. However, it is extremely important that you do not compromise yourself or others during the rescue operation e.g. run out in front of a car, jump head-first into shallow water or swim when there are large waves or strong currents.

Do something!

I have been in several situations where people have either been drowning or have been hurt in a serious car accident, and I have been happy for the knowledge I have acquired during the courses. It has made it possible for me to act on "autopilot" – quickly, efficiently and without hesitation, because the most important thing in CPR is to act.

> "A little less conversation – a little more action, please"
> ELVIS PRESLEY

Below is an excerpt from the latest guidelines regarding CPR as well as my personal recommendations. They cannot be substituted for a CPR course because a lot of details are omitted. For obvious reasons, reading cannot stand alone, but must be supplemented with essential practical experience such as heart massage and artificial respiration. Nevertheless, the main things are included in a simple and clear way, and rest assured that this can save lives. It is about making a world of difference.

Good advice on first aid

Check for consciousness and call emergency

The first thing you should do when you approach someone is to check whether the person is conscious. Speak to the person – say for instance "Hey, are you awake?", "Hello, are you okay?" or "Hello, are you well?". Do not yell or shout because in the worst-case scenario it can send the person into a state of shock. Shake his or her shoulder gently. If there is no response, the person is unconscious and you must immediately call for help. Ask someone else to dial 9-1-1 or do it on your own cell phone, turning on the loudspeaker, so you can talk on the phone without using your hands. This makes it possible to immediately begin lifesaving first aid.

Clear the airway

Make sure that the person is lying on his or her back and gently bend the head back and lift the chin to open the airways. This is extremely important, since many people suffocate in their own vomit, blood or on their tongue. Then remove any vomit or any other material from the mouth. If the person is not breathing, start CPR.

Start CPR (30:2)

Place your hands on top of each other in the middle of the chest, keep your elbows straight and position your shoulders directly above your hands to use the weight of your upper body to push hard down (1½ to 2 inches). Deliver 30 chest compressions fast, almost twice a second, with a frequency of 100 compressions per minute. After 30 compressions, give two rescue breaths which take approximately one second each. You can either blow through the nose or through the mouth, but remember to close the hole that you are not using in order to direct the air into the lungs. Do not blow too hard, as it can cause the person to throw up, but blow hard enough to make the chest of the person rise. If there are other people present, divide the tasks between you, so that one focuses on the compressions and the other on the rescue breaths.

Follow this rescue pattern (CPR with 30 compressions followed by two rescue breaths, that is a 30:2 ratio), since it provides the best blood circulation and the best distribution of oxygen in the unconscious person. Although the technique is called Cardio Pulmonary Resuscitation (CPR), it is primarily the brain you wish to save, and that is exactly what you do when you compress the heart and blow into the person's lungs. You are simply breathing for the unconscious person. Remember that you only absorb approximately one fourth of the oxygen you breathe. So even though the air you blow into the victim is "used", there is more than enough oxygen to oxygenate the blood for a short period of time.

Continue CPR until the person begins to breathe, an ambulance arrives and medics can take over, or until you no longer have the energy to continue. If the victim has suffered drowning or suffocation, it is recommended to begin CPR with five rescue breaths.

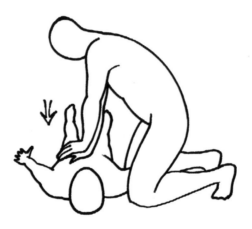

CPR is easy to learn and can save human lives.

Psychological first aid

As mentioned above, it is important that you do not shout or panic. Although the injured does not respond, it is possible that he/she can hear what you are saying because hearing is often one of the last senses to disappear. This is also true for people in coma. It is thus extremely important that you always speak with a clear and soothing voice, even when you talk with the Public Safety Answering Point on the phone or people standing by. Similarly, it is also important that people who help or are standing close to the injured, speak quietly and only in positive terms.

I have held and spoken reassuringly to a girl who was very badly injured after being hit by a taxi at high speed. During the course of events, a spectator started to scream that the girl was going to die unless the ambulance arrived soon. This only made matters worse. Be quiet or leave the place, if you do not intend to help.

Only use positive words and provide reassurance – say for instance: "I'll stay with you", "Help is on its way", "It's okay", etc. Do not say "You're not going to die", "It isn't that bad" or "Do not panic", because the brain is bound to focus on the words "die", "bad" or "panic". If the person is breathing, position him or her in the *recovery position*.

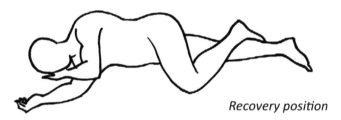

Recovery position

Place the injured person on the back. Pull the leg furthest away from you up in a right angle and roll the person towards yourself. Also pull the far arm and place the hand under the cheek.

Your calming breath

Use your breath to create peace, clarity and mental resources. Breathe deeply and slowly throughout the process and try wherever possible to relax the body so you do not tighten unnecessary muscles. You will thus work more efficiently and can aid for a longer time since heart-lung-rescue can be very demanding and tiring to perform for 5-10 minutes without a break. You will find out for yourself on your next CPR course.

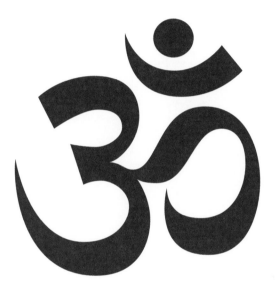

Your personal training program

As you may have noticed while reading this book, I believe one should act to retain or restore a healthy life. If you have a positive, cheerful and curious approach to training your body and mind, it will make it so much easier. Here are some ideas to how you can create your own training program that you can perform whenever and wherever you like.

It is entirely up to you as to what amount of time you wish to train, but as a starting point 10-20 minutes a day is just fine. If you get hooked on it and quickly feel the many positive changes the training provides, you can extend the program to 30-40 minutes or even a full hour, which may give you a very relaxing and thoroughly invigorating workout.

I will now offer you some recommendations on how to combine the exercises of the book through four basic phases. If you wish to do it in an entirely different way, it is up to you - switch between the exercises as you wish or add other exercises that you like.

As you will see, your training program consists of a couple of pages that are divided into four phases where you can enter your favorite exercises. In this way the training program becomes personal and is always at hand. Use a pencil – you can always create new programs as you become more experienced and acquire new ideas. There are a couple of pages dedicated to notes on your experiences and progress after your personal training program.

Phase 1: Mental and physical warm-up

If you start the exercises after a long day, it is a good idea to lie in the *Relaxed Position* and breathe calmly for a couple of minutes (p. 56). In this way your body and thoughts relax and mark the transition to your beautiful, calming and invigorating training program. If thoughts fly around in your head, a concentration and imagery exercise will benefit you greatly: *Gravitational Force*, *Sound Picture*, *Blue-Red Body*, *Ecstatic Joy* or *Paradise* (p. 58-59). That way you direct your thoughts to something positive and can more easily forget the negative thoughts of the day.

If you perform the exercises in the morning after a good night's sleep, or if your spirits are high and you are ready to go, just get started. Warm up your body and lungs with one or more of the following exercises:

Chest and shoulder stretch (p. 183)
Albatros (p. 184)
Sky stretch (p. 184)
Rag doll (p. 185)
Cat stretch (p. 239)
Wag your tail (p. 239)
Right angle (p. 240)
Plough pose (p. 240)
Child's pose (p. 241)
Maximum exhalation (p. 241)

Phase 2: Breathing exercises

When you want to train your breathing, you can select one or more of the following exercises:

1) General breathing exercises: *Neutral, Attention, Rhythm and pulse, Your Natural Rhythm* (p. 79-80).
2) Yogic breathing: *Yoga Breathing, Yoga Breathing with Abdominal Tension, Training the diaphragm* (p. 111-114).
3) Soothing pranayama – possibly with breath holding: *Victorious Breath, Alternate Nostril Breathing* (p. 151).

Start breathing with a 1:1 ratio of inhalation to exhalation.
    Afterwards you can exhale twice as long as you inhale.
    In time add a breath hold with empty as well as full lungs – inhale, breath hold, exhale, breath hold in the ratio 1:1:1:1. After weeks or months you can change this ratio or just do a breath hold on full lungs in the classic *Alternate Nostril Breathing* ratio of 1:4:2 (see the pranayama figure p. 153).
    It is extremely important that you do not breathe or hold your breath too long, because you have to avoid "gasping" for air.

1) Power training of the respiratory muscles (activating pranayama): *Brain Purification* (p. 154), *Bellows Breathing* (p. 154), *Natural chest press (Tarzan,* p. 186), *Artificial chest press (Snake,* p. 186).

2) Practice the three body locks during training: *Root Lock*, *Abdominal Lock*, *Throat Lock* (p. 242-243) If they are performed at the same time, they form *Great Lock* (*Maha Bandha*, p. 243).

Phase 3: Meditation and relaxation

When you want to meditate, the best position is a yoga posture where you sit with a straight back (p. 148-149). However, choose the position that suits you best. There are many kinds of meditation, but here we will boil it down to two types: One where the mind focuses on one particular thing e.g. your pulse, the sound of your breath, a thought or an object, and one where your thoughts passively observe and record everything in and around you, a kind of mindfulness meditation.

When you have finished, and your thoughts return to training, slowly lie down on your back in *Relaxed Position*. Close your eyes and perform a brief imagery or concentration exercise focusing on becoming completely relaxed – e.g. *Feel Your Heart* or *Beautiful Self-image* (p. 77-78). Take your time "returning" – wriggle your fingers and toes and open your eyes slowly.

Phase 4: Prayer

Close the session with a little inner prayer, perhaps with your palms together in front of your chest. You can also choose to end the session repeating three long Om (AAAUUUMMMMM).

Personal program for:_____

PHASE 1: MENTAL AND PHYSICAL WARM-UP (2-5 MINUTES)

_____

_____

_____

_____

_____

PHASE 2: BREATHING EXERCISES (5-10 MINUTES)

_____

_____

_____

_____

_____

_____

_____

_____

_____

_____

_____

_____

_____

_____

_____

PHASE 3: MEDITATION AND RELAXATION (2-10 MINUTES)

_____

_____

_____

_____

_____

PHASE 4: PRAYER (1-5 MINUTES)

_____

_____

_____

_____

_____

NOTES ON EXPERIENCES, THOUGHTS, IMPRESSIONS AND PROGRESS IN YOUR DAILY TRAINING

_____

_____

_____

_____

_____

_____

_____

_____

_____

_____

_____

_____

_____

_____

_____

_____

_____

_____

_____

_____

_____

_____

_____

_____

_____

_____

_____

_____

_____

_____

Disclaimer

Please note that this book is meant as a supplement and inspiration to your daily practice.

If you are in doubt or uncertain in regards to different exercises or any possible risks, you are advised to consult a professional teacher, instructor or physician.

It is the precise responsibility of the reader to understand the associated risks related to breathing and breath holding exercises. When performing breath holding in water (apnea), this should always be done with a professional instructor and all water activities should be done in pairs in order to maximize safety. Never dive alone.

Part of any human being's "safety & rescue" repertoire should be the ability to perform Cardio Pulmonary Resuscitation (CPR). You are recommended to join a specific course of theory and practice. Reading a book will not be sufficient. Seek instructions from a specialist in order to learn how to correctly manage an emergency procedure.

The reader bears the sole responsibility for adopting a behaviour which ensures safe activities. Any direct or indirect loss, injury or other incident, which may or may not happen after reading this book or information related to this book, is not the responsibility of author nor publisher.

Index

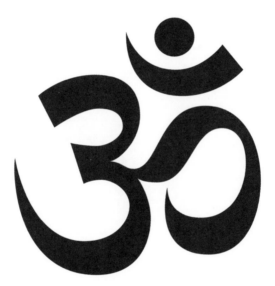

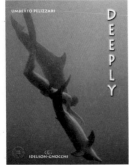

Deeply
by UMBERTO PELIZZARI
ISBN 1-928649-31-9
Hardcover: 224 pages
$ 50.00 - € 50,00

This book is not only an autobiography of Pelizzari, but also an incredible reflection on man's constant and irrepressible urge to exceed the limits imposed on him by nature, to experience new sensations and to go deep within himself in search of a freedom that knows no boundaries. Captivating images accompany a vivid narrative of the records and adventures that defined Pelizzari's life and sporting career: from the beginnings in the pool, to the discovery of his own ability, the training, the teamwork, acquaintances with the historic figures of the underwater world – such as Mayol and Maiorca – as well as the simple folk of the seas who live their lives in contact with the water, the victories, world records, and freedives in seas all over the world, and the encounters with the magnificent sea creatures that inhabit them. Page after page, Pelizzari relives the experience of his inner journey in the depths of the sea.

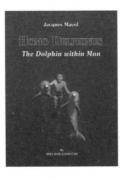

Homo Delphinus
The Dolphin Within Man
by JACQUES MAYOL
ISBN 192864903-3
Hardcover: 398 pages
$ 95.00 - € 75,00

The only book written about Ma spiritual connection to the se The term Homo Delphinus refe to individuals who are aquatic dolphin, share a love of the ocea Mayol believed that some people w be, within a couple of generatio capable of swimming at depths of 2 meters and holding their breath for to ten minutes.
This book is also a limited edition coffee-table size book includes mo than 300 pictures.

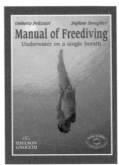

Manual of Freediving
Underwater on a single breath
by UMBERTO PELIZZARI and
STEFANO TOVAGLIERI
ISBN 192864927-0
Softcover: 366 pages
$ 39.50 - € 35,00

From theory to practice: the first e tirely illustrated and complete guide freediving.
The definitive guide, illustrated and to date, for the aspiring apneist. Fro theory to practice this manual will company the reader in the discovery c fascinating sport.
A manual that should not be missing from the itinerary of any diver (a neist or otherwise) who wishes to improve their techniques of respiratio swimming and diving whilst broadening knowledge and theory.
Dozens of exercises, illustrated with helpful sequences of pictures alle both student and instructors of apnea to follow a simple and effect teaching path. From the experience of two sportsmen, with years de cated to competitive and instructive apnea, finally a manual that uni theory with practical.

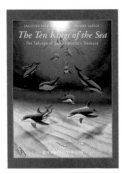

The Ten Kings of the Sea
Salvage of Santa Isabella's Treasure
by JACQUES and PIERRE MAYOL
ISBN 192864924-6
Softcover: 256 pages
$ 25.00 - € 19,50

A novel based on real discoveries and experiences made by Jacques Mayol around the world during his life who was dedicated to discovering the underwater secrets of the Sea.

forthcoming titles

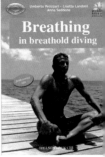

Breathing
in breathold diving
by UMBERTO PELIZZARI
LISETTA LANDONI
and ANNA SEDDONE
ISBN 192864932-7

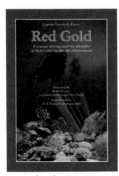

Red Gold
Extreme diving and the plunder of red coral in the Mediterranean
by Captain LEONARDO FUSCO
ISBN 192864929-7
Hardcover: 272 pages
$ 25.00 - € 30,00

Italian edition

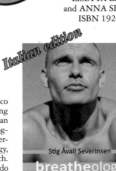

"In 1953, at Cape Spartivento, Leonardo Fusco made his first Aqua Lung dive, and everything changed. As spearfishing led Hans Hass to an underwater career of science, film and photography, so spearfishing led Leonardo to an underwater career of coral harvesting, marine biology, mixed gas technology and hyperbaric research. Diving to recover his lost speargun, Leonardo discovered a carpet of red coral, and his life took a whole new direction."

Leslie Leaney
co-founder of Historical Diving Society

www.redcoralsociety.org

Stig Åvall Severinsen
breatheology
the art of conscious breathing

Breatheology
the art of conscious breathing
by STIG ÅVALL SEVERINSEN